OVERVIEW-MAP KEY

THE BEST IN TENT CAMPING

NEW YORK STATE

Other books in the series:

THE BEST IN TENT CAMPING

A GUIDE FOR CAR CAMPERS WHO HATE RVs,
CONCRETE SLABS, AND LOUD PORTABLE STEREOS

NEW YORK STATE

Catharine Wells, Aaron Starmer,
and Timothy Starmer

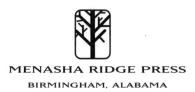

MENASHA RIDGE PRESS
BIRMINGHAM, ALABAMA

*For our parents, who fostered in us a love of the outdoors
and taught us to pitch our first tents.*

Copyright © 2007 by Catharine Wells, Aaron Starmer, and Timothy Starmer

Printed in the United States of America

Published by Menasha Ridge Press

Distributed by Publishers Group West

First edition, first printing

 Printed on recycled paper

Library of Congress Cataloging-in-Publication Data

Wells, Catharine, 1980—

    The best in tent camping, New York State: a guide for car campers who hate RVs, concrete slabs, and loud portable stereos/Catharine Wells, Aaron Starmer, and Timothy Starmer.—1st ed.

    p. cm.

Includes index.

    ISBN 13: 978-89732-641-4 (alk. paper)

    ISBN 10: 0-89732-641-5 (alk. paper)

    1. Camp sites, facilities, etc.—New York (State)—Directories. 2. Camping—New York (State)—Guidebooks. 3. New York (State)—Guidebooks. I. Starmer, Aaron, 1976— II. Starmer, Timothy, 1975— III. Title.

    GV194.N64W45 2007

    796.5409747—dc22

    2007001707

Cover and text design by Ian Szymkowiak, Palace Press International, Inc.

Cover photograph by Jonathan Sherrill/Alamy

Cartography by Catharine Wells, Aaron Starmer, Timothy Starmer, and Jennie Zehmer

Indexing by Rich Carlson

Menasha Ridge Press

P.O. Box 43673

Birmingham, Alabama 35243

www.menasharidge.com

TABLE OF CONTENTS

ADIRONDACKS 85

THOUSAND ISLANDS 141

FINGER LAKES 149

WESTERN NEW YORK 165

APPENDIXES AND INDEX 175

OUR TOP 5
NEW YORK STATE
CAMPGROUNDS

1. **FORKED LAKE**
   (PROFILE 29, ADIRONDACKS, PAGE 104)
2. **WATCH HILL**
   (PROFILE 3, LONG ISLAND, PAGE 20)
3. **MARY ISLAND STATE PARK**
   (PROFILE 41, THOUSAND ISLANDS, PAGE 142)
4. **BUCK POND**
   (PROFILE 26, ADIRONDACKS, PAGE 95)
5. **LITTLE POND**
   (PROFILE 7, CATSKILLS AND HUDSON VALLEY, PAGE 34)

ACKNOWLEDGMENTS

WE WOULD LIKE TO THANK Russell Helms, Ritchey Halphen, and the whole gang at Menasha Ridge Press, whose helpful input and confidence in our abilities saw this book through to completion. We started our project with a visit to Watch Hill Campground in Long Island, where Marybeth and the staff of the camping concession as well as the rangers of the Fire Island National Seashore confirmed our hope that this project would be hard work but also a lot of fun. Tom Folts and the welcoming staff at the New York State Department of Environmental Conservation made our visits to the Adirondacks and the Catskills especially memorable. The many workers in the New York state-park system always answered our questions with a smile and trusted us enough to set us loose in their facilities with our cameras and notebooks. Finally, we would like to thank our employers for happily tolerating our working vacations, and our friends and families who listened to us blather on about our adventures.

PREFACE

WE HAVE ALWAYS BEEN TENT CAMPERS. From summer nights in the backyard, to family odysseys through the wilds of the Northeast, to trips abroad with pounds of gear strapped to our backs, tent camping has been an essential part of our lives. Did we ever expect to write a book about tent camping? Admittedly, no. But as we loaded up our cars, preparing to take on the task of deciding which 50 places in New York are the best to pitch a tent, we knew we were shouldering a certain responsibility. Choosing a campground can be a frustrating endeavor, a game of dice where you hope your roll won't put you in a glorified parking lot, breathing in exhaust fumes and inserting earplugs to make it through the night. We had to do a good job, because this is a book we ourselves would want to use, many times over.

But New York is a deceptively large state. And there are plenty of campgrounds to go around. Quite early in the project, we discovered we wouldn't have a problem finding worthy candidates. Like coaches, we were faced with the unenviable duty of making cuts. In the Adirondack and Catskill mountains alone, there are 52 state-run campgrounds, to say nothing of privately run facilities and innumerable hike-in sites. We crisscrossed the state, burning up gas, jotting down pages of notes, and, of course, pitching our tents. To our surprise, each campground we visited was quite distinct, and therefore this wouldn't be just a matter of flipping coins.

So we set up a system. We divided the state into seven regions, divisions native New Yorkers will find familiar. We made it a point to provide an even distribution of camping choices. If there were a handful of campgrounds within a few miles of each other, we would choose only the best of the bunch. We favored campgrounds near lakes, rivers, or oceans; and surroundings that were either brimming with recreational opportunities or reproduced the quiet thrill of backcountry camping, albeit with the occasional comfort station. Unless the settings were truly spectacular, we shunned campgrounds where RVs were in the majority and reservations were as hard to obtain as those at a fancy restaurant. In short, we chose the campgrounds where we, at different stages in our lives, might find ourselves enjoying a night under the stars.

Maybe you won't find your favorite childhood campground in this book. Hopefully, what you will find are some overlooked campgrounds, located in vibrant (historically, culturally, and naturally) corners of New York. And ideally, you'll get out there to explore as many as possible. We've seen them all, and we can't wait for the next camping season to begin.

—Catharine Wells, Aaron Starmer, and Timothy Starmer

ABOUT THE AUTHORS

CATHARINE WELLS was born on Cape Cod, and her parents' many moves throughout the Northeast inspired her lifelong wanderlust. She pitched her first tent as a Girl Scout in Penn's Woods. Backpacking trips during college took her as far as Australia, Thailand, and Costa Rica. Her favorite camping spots are usually near the water, such as Flamenco Beach in Puerto Rico and Watch Hill on Fire Island. Currently a book editor in New York City, Cate often loads up her pack and escapes into the wilderness on weekends. She always makes sure her first-aid kit contains heaps of bandages, plenty of sunscreen, and a corkscrew for emergencies.

Growing up outside of Syracuse, **AARON STARMER** spent his childhood exploring the wilds of central New York. As a graduation present from Drew University, he received a tent, which has become his favorite accommodation on trips around the country. He has pitched it on the rim of the Grand Canyon, in the shadow of the Watchman at Zion National Park, deep in the woods of the Great Smoky Mountains, and on Flamenco Beach in Culebra, Puerto Rico. For years he has worked in New York City as an editor for Longitude Books, a bookseller specializing in recommended reading for travelers. His writing has appeared in *McSweeney's* and other humor publications. Currently a resident of Hoboken, New Jersey, he hopes to write, travel, and pitch that tent more with each coming year.

TIM STARMER has always been an outdoor enthusiast and spent most of his childhood seeking out remote and wild areas whenever possible. During a brief hiatus from Brown University during 1997, he drove across the United States for six weeks, camping the entire way. Along the way he explored many of the West's national and state parks, including Canyonlands, Yellowstone, Arches, Bryce Canyon—he even braved pitching a tent among the mosquito swarms in Badlands National Park. At the trip's conclusion, he headed down to Australia, where he backpacked for a few months exploring the eastern Outback, the Great Barrier Reef, and the caves of Tasmania, as well as traversing the Tasmanian World Heritage Area along the Overland Track. Tim currently works in upstate New York as a timber framer and can still be found exploring the wilds whenever possible.

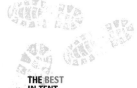

THE BEST IN TENT CAMPING

NEW YORK STATE

INTRODUCTION

WHEN MOST PEOPLE HEAR THE WORDS "New York," they naturally think of the "Big Apple." While New York City is undoubtedly an important part of the state, there's so much beyond its borders, especially for those interested in the outdoors. Whether you think that Upstate begins at the edge of the five boroughs or includes Long Island, you cannot deny that wilderness abounds in New York state. From the Great Lakes to the Atlantic Ocean, from the Adirondack Mountains to the Catskills, from the St. Lawrence River to the Hudson, tent campers wishing to explore the state have a wide variety of campgrounds from which to choose. Here we highlight the 50 best. Eschewing the noisy, the busy, the overbooked, and the badly maintained, we have chosen peaceful and scenic campgrounds by lakes, on islands, near beaches, along rivers, and deep in the woods.

There are no national parks in New York state, but its state-park system is one of the country's finest. Almost all of the campgrounds featured in this book are state-run and range in size from a dozen sites to more than 200. Most are accessible by car, but a handful of boat-only and walk-in sites are included for the more adventurous. The Adirondack and Catskills parks are run by the New York State Department of Environmental Conservation, whereas others are run by the New York State Office of Parks, Recreation and Historic Preservation.

The gem of the state's recreation opportunities is easy to spot on a map—a huge patch of green that covers one-fifth of the state, the **Adirondack Park**. Conservation of this 6-million-acre wilderness has been in effect since 1892, earlier than the creation of almost all the major national parks in the American West. Age is not the only trump card Adirondack Park can play—it is larger than Yellowstone, Glacier, Grand Canyon, and Everglades national parks combined. Parcels of state-owned "forever wild" forest preserve are interspersed with private lands, providing an experience similar to some of the largest parks in Europe. This combination is perfect for tent campers, as the wilderness is all around you, but supplies and other recreational opportunities are always near. The High Peaks region of the Adirondacks attracts avid hikers, and the innumerable lakes offer something for all types of boats, from large motorboats on Lake George to canoes and kayaks in the St. Regis Canoe Wilderness.

Both the Catskills and the Hudson Valley have been greatly influenced by their proximity to New York City. **Catskill Park** is similar to the Adirondacks in its combination of public and private lands and conservation policies, but these oldest mountains in the state have been known throughout recent history as a playground for the city's wealthy. The Hudson Valley, to the east of the Catskills, is home to luxurious estates and, of course, the famed river, an essential lifeline which for years has pumped goods and travelers to and from the bustling metropolis at its mouth.

The heart of New York is the history-rich **Central**, or **Leatherstocking**, region. In addition to Colonial and Revolutionary War sites, visitors will find Howe Caverns and the Baseball Hall of Fame. We've combined this area with the **Saratoga-Capital** region, home to races of two types: political ones in the capital city of Albany, and annual horse races in Saratoga Springs.

The **Finger Lakes,** with their long, thin bodies of water and nearby rolling hills, are remnants from the Ice Ages. Dramatic gorges and waterfalls attract hikers throughout the year, but especially in the spring as floodwaters surge through carved rock walls, and in the fall, when it's a leaf-peeping paradise. Award-winning wineries are more-recent additions that attract plenty of tourists, including the occasional tent camper.

Long Island is where you will find camping on and near the Atlantic Ocean, perfect for surf-fishermen and sun-worshipers alike. It may be surprising, but good tent camping can be found not far from the glamorous Hamptons. For a truly unique experience, take the ferry to the car-free Fire Island and its national seashore and pitch your tent in the sand.

Fishing, boating, and water sports attract many visitors to the vacation wonderland known as the **Thousand Islands** on the St. Lawrence River. Getting lost among the myriad islands that form the border between the United States and Canada is a common cruising adventure here. Some people prefer to just relax on the shore and watch ocean liners chug along from America's heartland toward the Atlantic Ocean.

In **Western New York,** the wide shores of Lake Erie flow over Niagara Falls into Lake Ontario. It is also where you'll find the Allegheny Mountains and Allegany State Park, the largest park run by the state's Office of Parks, Recreation and Historic Preservation. Don't miss the deep-cut gorge often referred to as "Grand Canyon of the East," found in Letchworth State Park.

Read on, and hopefully you'll see there is so much more in the state than the skyscrapers and bustling streets of Manhattan. Most state natives already know it is an outdoor destination to rival any in the country. But we believe even the most seasoned New York camper will find some new places to explore. Pitch a tent at any of the campgrounds we feature, and you'll discover even more reasons to love New York.

But before embarking on a trip, take time to prepare. Many of the best tent campgrounds are a fair distance from the civilized world, and you want to be enjoying yourself rather than making supply or gear runs. Call ahead and ask for a park map, brochure, or other information to help you plan your trip. Visit the campground's Web site (listed for each destination in this book under **Key Information**). Make reservations wherever applicable, especially at popular state parks. Ask questions. Ask more questions. The more questions you ask, the fewer surprises you will get. There are other times, however, when you'll want to grab your gear and this book, hop in the car, and just wing it. This can be an adventure in its own right.

RESERVATIONS

For all but two of the campgrounds listed in this book (Sears Bellows County Park and Watch Hill Campground), reservations should be placed through **ReserveAmerica**, a convenient online and telephone service that lets you choose from available sites and pay by credit card up to nine months in advance of your stay. For more information, call (800) 456-2267 or visit **www.reserveamerica.com**.

THE OVERVIEW MAP AND OVERVIEW-MAP KEY

Use the overview map on the inside front cover to assess the exact location of each campground. The campground's number appears not only on the overview map but also on the map key facing the overview map, in the table of contents, and on the profile's first page.

The book is organized by region, as indicated in the table of contents. A map legend that details the symbols found on the campground layout maps appears on the inside back cover.

CAMPGROUND-LAYOUT MAPS

Each profile contains a detailed campground-layout map that provides an overhead look at campground sites, internal roads, facilities, and other key items. Each campground entrance's GPS coordinates are included with each profile.

GPS COORDINATES

This book also includes GPS coordinates for each campground profile in two formats: Universal Transverse Mercator (UTM) and latitude–longitude. Latitude–longitude coordinates tell you where you are by locating a point west (latitude) of the 0° meridian line that passes through Greenwich, England, and north or south of the 0° (longitude) line that belts the Earth, aka the Equator.

Topographic maps show latitude and longitude as well as UTM grid lines. Known as UTM coordinates, the numbers index a specific point using a grid method. The survey datum used to arrive at the coordinates in this book is WGS84 (versus NAD27 or WGS83). For readers who own a GPS unit, whether handheld or onboard a vehicle, the latitude–longitude or UTM coordinates may be entered into the GPS unit (just make sure your unit is set to navigate using WGS84 datum). Now you can navigate directly to the campground. (Coordinates that do not lead directly to a campground entrance, such as those for a general state-park entrance or a boat landing, have been noted as such.)

That said, however, readers can easily find all campgrounds in this book by using the directions given and the campground layout map, which shows at least one major road leading into the area. But for those who enjoy using the latest GPS technology to navigate, the necessary data have been provided. A brief explanation of the UTM coordinates for Clarence Fahnestock Memorial State Park (page 28), follows:

PARK ENTRANCE:
UTM Zone (WGS84)   18T
Easting   598124
Northing   4591124

Latitude   N 41°27'57"
Longitude   W 73°49'30"

The UTM zone number **18** refers to one of the 60 vertical zones of the Universal Transverse Mercator (UTM) projection. Each zone is 6 degrees wide. The UTM zone letter **T** refers to one of the 20 horizontal zones that span from 80 degrees South to 84 degrees North. The easting number **598124** indicates in meters how far east or west a point is from the central meridian of the zone. Increasing easting coordinates on a topographic map or on your GPS screen indicate that you are moving east; decreasing easting coordinates indicate you are moving west. The northing number **4591124** references in meters how far you are from the equator. Above and below the equator, increasing northing coordinates indicate you are traveling north; decreasing northing coordinates indicate you are traveling south.

To learn more about how to enhance your outdoor experiences with GPS technology, refer to *GPS Outdoors: A Practical Guide for Outdoor Enthusiasts* (Menasha Ridge Press).

THE CAMPGROUND PROFILE

In addition to maps, each profile contains a concise but informative narrative of the campground, as well as individual sites. This descriptive text is enhanced with four helpful sidebars: **Ratings, Key Information, Getting There** (accurate driving directions that lead you to the campground from the nearest major roadway), and **GPS Coordinates.** On the first page of each profile is a Ratings box:

THE RATING SYSTEM

This book includes a rating system for New York state's 50 best tent campgrounds. Certain campground attributes—beauty, privacy, spaciousness, quiet, security, and cleanliness—are ranked using a five-star system. A low rating in one or two areas, especially privacy and spaciousness, was not necessarily grounds for exclusion from this book. In some cases, the nature of the terrain just doesn't allow for big, private sites, yet the campground still may be well worth a visit. This system should help you find what you are looking for.

BEAUTY In the best campgrounds, the fluid shapes and elements of nature—flora, water, land, and sky—have melded to create locales that seem to have been made for tent camping. The best sites are so attractive you may be tempted not to leave your outdoor home. A little site work to make the scenic area camper friendly is acceptable, but too many reminders of civilization eliminated many a campground from inclusion in this book.

PRIVACY A little understory goes a long way toward making you comfortable once you've picked your site for the night. There is a trend toward planting natural borders between campsites if the borders don't already exist. With some trees or brush to define the sites, everyone has personal space, so you can go about the pleasures of tent camping without minding your neighbors.

SPACIOUSNESS This attribute can be very important, depending on how much of a gearhead you are and the size of your group. Campers with family-style tents need a large, flat spot on which to pitch their tent, but still need to be able to get to the ice chest to prepare food while not getting burned by the fire ring. Gearheads need adequate space to show off all their stuff to passersby. We just want enough room to keep our bedroom, den, and kitchen separate.

QUIET The music of the mountains, rivers, and land between—the singing birds, rushing streams, and wind whooshing through the trees—includes the kinds of noises tent campers associate with being in New York. In concert, they camouflage the sounds you don't want to hear—autos coming and going, loud neighbors, and so on.

SECURITY Campground security is relative. A remote campground with no civilization nearby is usually safe, but don't tempt potential thieves by leaving your valuables out for all to see. Use common sense and go with your instinct. Campground hosts are wonderful to have around, and state parks with locked gates are ideal for security. Get to know your neighbors and, when possible, develop a buddy system for watching each other's belongings.

CLEANLINESS Nothing will sabotage a scenic campground like trash. Most of the campgrounds in this guidebook are clean. More-rustic campgrounds—our favorites—usually receive less maintenance. Busy weekends and holidays will show their effects; however, don't let a little litter spoil your good time. Help clean up, and think of it as doing your part for New York's natural environment.

WEATHER

Spring is the most variable season. During March, you'll find your first signs of rebirth in the lowlands, yet trees in the high country may not be fully leafed out until June. Both winter- and summerlike weather can occur in spring. As summer approaches, the strong fronts weaken, and thunderstorms and haze become more frequent. Summertime rainy days can be cool. In fall, continental fronts once again sweep through, clearing the air and bringing warm days and cool nights, though rain is always possible.

The first snows of winter usually arrive in November, and snow falls intermittently through April. About 40 to 120 inches of snow can fall during this time. Expect to incur entire days of below-freezing weather, though temperatures may range from mild to bitterly cold.

FIRST-AID KIT

A useful first-aid kit may contain more items than you might think necessary. These are just the basics. Prepackaged kits in waterproof bags (Atwater Carey and Adventure Medical make them) are available. As a preventive measure, take along sunscreen and insect repellent. Even though quite a few items are listed here, they pack down into a small space:

Ace bandages or Spenco joint wraps

Adhesive bandages, such as Band-Aids

Antibiotic ointment (Neosporin or the generic equivalent)

Antiseptic or disinfectant, such as Betadine or hydrogen peroxide

Aspirin or acetaminophen

Benadryl or the generic equivalent, diphenhydramine (in case of allergic reactions)

Butterfly-closure bandages

Epinephrine in a prefilled syringe (for people known to have severe allergic reactions to such things as bee stings)

Gauze (one roll)

Gauze compress pads (six 4- x 4-inch pads)

Matches or pocket lighter

Moleskin/Spenco "Second Skin"

Waterproof first-aid tape

Whistle (it's more effective in signaling rescuers than your voice)

ANIMAL AND PLANT HAZARDS

SNAKES New York has a variety of snakes—including garter, milk, and water snakes—most of which are benign. Timber rattlesnakes, northern copperheads, and eastern massasauga rattlesnakes are the exceptions, though they primarily dwell in very remote areas.

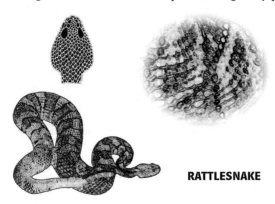

RATTLESNAKE

According to the state's Department of Environmental Conservation, the massasauga inhabits two isolated marshy areas: one near Syracuse and the other near Rochester. The copperhead is found mostly along the Hudson Valley but is generally absent from the Catskills. The timber rattlesnake is the most widely dispersed of the three and is found in rugged deciduous forests along the southern edge of the state and up into the eastern Adirondacks. Encounters with any of these species are very rare.

When hiking, stick to well-used trails, and wear over-the-ankle boots and loose-fitting long pants. Rattlesnakes like to bask in the sun and won't bite unless threatened. Don't step or put your hands where you can't see, and avoid wandering in the dark. Step on logs and rocks, never over them (so you can see any snakes on the other side), and be careful when climbing rocks or gathering firewood. Avoid walking through dense brush or willow thickets. Hibernation season is October through April.

TICKS Ticks are often found on brush and tall grass waiting to hitch a ride on a warm-blooded passerby. Adult ticks are most active in the New York between April and May and again between October and November. Among the local varieties of ticks, the black-legged tick, commonly called the deer tick, is the primary carrier of Lyme disease. (In general, deer ticks are much smaller than wood, or dog, ticks—about the size of a freckle—and are uniformly dark in color, whereas wood ticks usually have white spots.)

You can use several strategies to reduce your chances of a tick bite. Some people choose to wear light-colored clothing, so ticks can be spotted before they make it to the skin. Most important, be sure to visually check your hair, the back of your neck, your armpits, and your socks at the end of the hike. During your posthike shower, take a moment to do a more-complete body check. For ticks that are already embedded, removal with sharp tweezers is best: place them as close to skin as possible and gently rotate out, taking care not to squeeze the tick. Use disinfectant solution on the wound. To be on the safe side, you may want to visit a physician as soon as possible and follow his or her advice on taking a course of antibiotics to ward off a possible case of Lyme disease. (It takes a few hours for an embedded carrier tick to infect the person it's bitten.)

POISON IVY, OAK, AND SUMAC

Recognizing and avoiding these three plants are the most effective ways to prevent the painful, itchy rashes associated with them. Poison ivy occurs as a vine or groundcover, 3 leaflets to a leaf; poison oak occurs as either a vine or shrub, also with 3 leaflets; and poison sumac flourishes in swampland, each leaf having 7 to 13 leaflets. Urushiol, the oil in the sap of these plants, is responsible for the rash. Remember that all parts of the plant contain the oil and you can get a reaction even from the leafless plant in winter. Within 14 hours of exposure, raised lines and/or blisters will appear on the affected area, accompanied by a terrible itch.

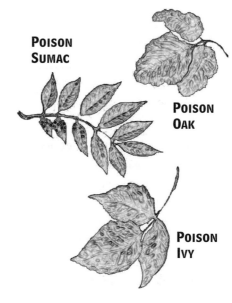

POISON SUMAC

POISON OAK

POISON IVY

Refrain from scratching, because bacteria under your fingernails can cause an infection. Wash and dry the rash thoroughly, applying a lotion containing calamine to help dry out the rash. If itching or blistering is severe, seek medical attention. If you do come into contact with one of these plants, remember that oil-contaminated clothes, pets, or hiking gear can easily cause an irritating rash on you or someone else, so wash not only any exposed parts of your body but also clothes, gear, and pets.

BLACK BEARS Black bears are found throughout New York state, but are most frequently encountered in the Adirondacks and occasionally in the Catskills. Though attacks by black bears are virtually unheard of, a bear tearing up your gear or rummaging about outside your tent will give anyone a start. If you encounter a bear at your campsite or while hiking, remain calm and never run away. Make loud noises to scare off the bear and back away slowly. In primitive and remote areas, assume that bears are present; in more-developed sites, ask the park staff about the current bear situation. Most encounters are food-related, as bears have an exceptional sense of smell and will eat anything and everything. A clean site, combined with care and caution, will keep these foragers away from your campsite. Store all food, cooking equipment, and garbage in tightly sealed containers placed well away from your tent. In remote areas or those with recent bear activity, store all items in storage lockers, bear canisters, or suspend in a sack 12 feet above the ground, 6 feet below branches, and 12 feet from neighboring trees. Make sure that your site is clean, and never leave food unattended. Clean your utensils and cooking equipment at least 100 feet from your site and never dump uneaten food on the ground. Do not bring food into your tent and do not sleep in clothes worn while preparing food. Generally, proper food preparation and garbage disposal will help maintain a pristine wilderness, the safety of bears and other wildlife, and an enjoyable camping experience for everyone.

TIPS FOR A HAPPY CAMPING TRIP

There is nothing worse than a bad camping trip, especially because it is so easy to have a great time. To assist with making your outing a happy one, here are some pointers:

- **RESERVE YOUR SITE AHEAD OF TIME,** especially if it's a weekend, a holiday, or if the campground is wildly popular. Many prime campgrounds require at least a six-month lead time on reservations. Check before you go.

- **PICK YOUR CAMPING BUDDIES WISELY.** A family trip is pretty straight-forward, but you may want to reconsider including grumpy Uncle Fred, who doesn't like bugs, sunshine, or marshmallows. After you know who's going, make sure that everyone is on the same page regarding expectations of difficulty (amenities or the lack thereof, physical exertion, and so on), sleeping arrange-ments, and food requirements.

- **DON'T DUPLICATE EQUIPMENT** such as cooking pots and lanterns among campers in your party. Carry what you need to have a good time, but don't turn the trip into a major moving experience.

- **DRESS FOR THE SEASON.** Educate yourself on the temperature highs and lows of the specific area you plan to visit. It may be warm at night in the summer in your backyard, but up in the mountains it will be quite chilly.

- **PITCH YOUR TENT ON A LEVEL SURFACE,** preferably one covered with leaves, pine straw, or grass. Use a tarp or specially designed footprint to thwart ground moisture and to protect the tent floor. Do a little site maintenance, such as picking up the small rocks and sticks that can damage your tent floor and make sleep uncomfortable. If you have a separate tent rain fly but don't think you'll need it, keep it rolled up at the base of the tent in case it starts raining at midnight.

- **IF YOU ARE NOT COMFORTABLE SLEEPING ON THE GROUND, TAKE A SLEEPING PAD** with you that is full-length and thicker than you think you might need. This will not only keep your hips from aching on hard ground, but will also help keep you warm. A wide range of thin, light, inflatable pads is available at camping stores today, and these are a much better choice than home air mattresses, which conduct heat away from the body and tend to deflate during the night.

- **IF YOU'RE NOT HIKING IN TO A PRIMITIVE CAMPSITE,** there is no real need to skimp on food due to weight. Plan tasty meals and bring everything you will need to prepare, cook, eat, and clean up.

- **IF YOU TEND TO USE THE BATHROOM MULTIPLE TIMES AT NIGHT,** you should plan ahead. Leaving a warm sleeping bag and stumbling around in the dark to find the restroom, whether it be a pit toilet, a fully plumbed comfort station, or just the woods, is not fun. Keep a flashlight and any other accoutrements you may need by the tent door and know exactly where to head in the dark.

- **STANDING DEAD TREES AND STORM-DAMAGED LIVING TREES CAN POSE A REAL HAZARD** to tent campers. These trees may have loose or broken limbs that could fall at any time. When choosing a campsite or even just a spot to rest during a hike, look up.

CAMPING ETIQUETTE

Camping experiences can vary wildly depending on a variety of factors, such as weather, preparedness, fellow campers, and time of year. Here are a few tips on how to create good vibes with fellow campers and wildlife you encounter.

- **OBTAIN ALL PERMITS AND AUTHORIZATION AS REQUIRED.** Make sure you check in, pay your fee, and mark your site as directed. Don't make the mistake of grabbing a seemingly empty site that looks more appealing than your site. It could be reserved. If you're unhappy with the site you've selected, check with the campground host for other options.

- **LEAVE ONLY FOOTPRINTS.** Be sensitive to the ground beneath you. Be sure to place all garbage in designated receptacles or pack it out if none is available. No one likes to see the trash someone else has left behind.

- **NEVER SPOOK ANIMALS.** It's common for animals to wander through campsites, where they may be accustomed to the presence of humans (and our food). An unannounced approach, a sudden movement, or a loud noise startles most animals. A surprised animal can be dangerous to you, to others, and to themselves. Give them plenty of space.

- **PLAN AHEAD.** Know your equipment, your ability, and the area where you are camping—and prepare accordingly. Be self-sufficient at all times; carry necessary supplies for changes in weather or other conditions. A well-executed trip is a satisfaction to you and to others.

- **BE COURTEOUS TO OTHER CAMPERS,** hikers, bikers, and others you encounter. If you run into the owner of a large RV, don't panic. Just wave, feign eye contact, and then walk slowly away.

- **STRICTLY FOLLOW THE CAMPGROUND'S RULES** regarding the building of fires. Never burn trash. Trash smoke smells horrible, and trash debris in a fire pit or grill is unsightly.

BACKCOUNTRY-CAMPING ADVICE

A permit is not required before entering the backcountry to camp in the Adirondacks and Catskills. However, you should practice low-impact camping. Adhere to the adages "Pack it in, pack it out" and "Take only pictures, leave only footprints." Practice leave-no-trace camping ethics while in the backcountry.

Open fires are permitted except during dry times when the forest service may issue a fire ban. Backpacking stoves are strongly encouraged. You are required to hang your food away from bears and other animals to prevent them from becoming introduced to (and dependent on) human food. Wildlife learns to associate backpacks and backpackers with easy food sources, thereby influencing its behavior.

Solid human waste must be buried in a hole at least three inches deep and at least 200 feet away from trails and water sources; a trowel is basic backpacking equipment.

Following the above guidelines will increase your chances for a pleasant, safe, and low-impact interaction with nature.

VENTURING AWAY FROM THE CAMPGROUND

If you go for a hike, bike, or other excursion into the wilderness, here are some tips:

- **ALWAYS CARRY FOOD AND WATER,** whether you are planning to go overnight or not. Food will give you energy, help keep you warm, and sustain you in an emergency until help arrives. Bring potable water or treat water by boiling or filtering before drinking from a lake or stream.

- **STAY ON DESIGNATED TRAILS.** Most hikers get lost when they leave the trail. Even on the most clearly marked trails, there is usually a point where you have to stop and consider which direction to head. If you become disoriented, don't panic. As soon as you think you may be off-track, stop, assess your current direction, and then retrace your steps back to the point where you went awry. If you have absolutely no idea how to continue, return to the trailhead the way you came in. Should you become completely lost and have no idea of how to return to the trailhead, remaining in place along the trail and waiting for help is most often the best option for adults and always the best option for children.

- **BE ESPECIALLY CAREFUL WHEN CROSSING STREAMS.** Whether you are fording the stream or crossing on a log, make every step count. If you have any doubt about maintaining your balance on a log, go ahead and ford the stream instead. When fording a stream, use a trekking pole or stout stick for balance and face upstream as you cross. If a stream seems too deep to ford, turn back. Whatever is on the other side is not worth risking your life.

THE BEST IN TENT CAMPING
NEW YORK STATE

- **BE CAREFUL AT OVERLOOKS.** Although these areas may provide spectacular views, they are potentially hazardous. Stay back from the edge of outcrops and be absolutely sure of your footing: a misstep can mean a nasty and possibly fatal fall.

- **KNOW THE SYMPTOMS OF HYPOTHERMIA.** Shivering and forgetfulness are the two most common indicators of this insidious killer. Hypothermia can occur at any elevation, even in the summer. Wearing cotton clothing puts you especially at risk, because cotton, when wet, wicks heat away from the body. To prevent hypothermia, dress in layers using synthetic clothing for insulation, use a cap and gloves to reduce heat loss, and protect yourself with waterproof, breathable outerwear. If symptoms arise, get the victim to shelter, a fire, hot liquids, and dry clothes or a dry sleeping bag.

- **TAKE ALONG YOUR BRAIN.** A cool, calculating mind is the single most important piece of equipment you'll ever need on the trail. Think before you act. Watch your step. Plan ahead. Avoiding accidents before they happen is the best recipe for a rewarding and relaxing hike.

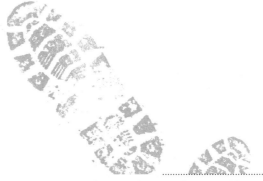
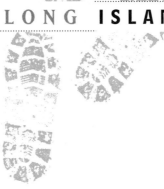

LONG ISLAND

1
HECKSCHER STATE PARK

IF THE WIDE, GRASSY FIELDS of Heckscher State Park bring to mind an elegant country estate, then you have already discovered something about its history. In the late 1800s, the eccentric and reclusive George C. Taylor purchased the property, built a large manor house on it, and dotted the land with a series of outbuildings. He then filled the woods with white-tailed deer (the descendants of which are often seen today), game birds, peacocks, and even a herd of elk. Upon Taylor's death, legal disputes over ownership complicated matters, and the land lay unused for years. Thanks in part to donations from August Heckscher, the Long Island State Park Commission finally purchased the area in 1929. The campground was established only a few years later.

With Nicoll Bay on its eastern edge and the Great South Bay forming its southern boundary, Heckscher is largely bordered by water. Fewer than 50 miles from New York City, it is a convenient getaway for many city visitors who create a very high volume of day-users. The park, located at the end of the aptly named Heckscher State Parkway, has well-maintained, clean, and secure facilities. Park police are a common site; day visitors are shuffled out at sundown, and the main campground gate closes at 10 p.m. In addition, campers are not allowed in areas outside the campground after sundown.

The campground is nestled in the woods, set off from Heckscher Parkway loop by an open field. As you enter, look for the campground office on your right. Arranged in a simple rectangle, and divided into four rows, the sites are closely spaced, but nicely shaded, well manicured, and flat. One large comfort station serves the campground in the center.

Use the grill for cooking. Other fires are permitted only in metal-bottom containers that the camper must bring. Each basic site features a cement platform, and

> *If we have one piece of advice, it's this: bring a bike.*

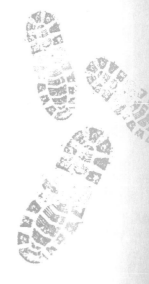

RATINGS

Beauty: ✩ ✩ ✩
Privacy: ✩ ✩
Quiet: ✩ ✩
Cleanliness: ✩ ✩ ✩ ✩
Security: ✩ ✩ ✩ ✩ ✩
Spaciousness: ✩ ✩

ADDRESS: P.O. Box 160 Heckscher State Parkway East Islip, NY 11730

OPERATED BY: New York State Office of Parks, Recreation and Historic Preservation

INFORMATION: (631) 581-2100; nysparks.state.ny.us

OPEN: Late May–early September

SITES: 69

EACH SITE HAS: Picnic table and grill

ASSIGNMENT: Choose from available sites or reservations

REGISTRATION: On arrival

FACILITIES: Water, flush toilets, pay phone, hot showers

PARKING: At site, 1 vehicle maximum, 1 additional at separate lot

FEE: $14/night (plus $3/night on Friday, Saturday, and holidays)

ELEVATION: 28 feet

RESTRICTIONS: *Pets:* Not allowed
Fires: In grill or approved container only
Alcohol: At site
Vehicles: No maximum
Other: Quiet hours 10 p.m.–7 a.m.
Reservations: 2-night stay required

RVs (limited to less than 11 feet high) are not an uncommon sight. However, there are no electrical or water hookups and quiet hours (when generators must be turned off) are strictly enforced. At the back of the far loop, you will find the quietest sites, with 67 and 68 being the most spacious. Although there is little to do in the campground itself, activities are organized in the summer for children, and families find it an ideal place to find respite from the more trafficked sections of the park.

If we have one piece of advice, it is this: bring a bike. The flat, bike-friendly trails offer fantastic riding opportunities for the casual cyclist. When we visited, we envied everyone who was exploring the park on two wheels. At 1,679 acres, Heckscher is difficult to see in its entirety on foot. And who would want to only see the park through the frame of a car window?

Bikers will be pleased, but hikers are certainly not forgotten. The park is home to 20 miles of trails, some of which connect the main park amenities. Follow the Greenbelt Trail southeast directly from the campground for a lovely walk along the edge of Nicoll Bay, ending at the Overlook Bathing Area on the Great South Bay. Following the same trail north takes you out of the park, leading eventually to Sunken Meadow State Park on Long Island Sound. At 32 miles one-way, you can choose to hike as far out and back as your feet and time allow.

Some of the many other facilities at Heckscher include a swimming pool, two sandy bathing areas (West Bathing Area and the previously mentioned Overlook) for swimming, playgrounds, softball and soccer fields, a boat basin and small boat launching ramp, bridle paths, and a sailing beach (popular with windsurfers). Picnic areas and pavilions are set back from the water, but a refreshment stand and first-aid station are handy for beachgoers. The sheer number of parking fields testifies to the multitude of visitors at the park, with eight separate parking areas available. In the course of a year, the park usually expects more than 1 million people to pass through its gates.

If you are looking to venture farther afield, campers can use their passes for free entrance into

MAP

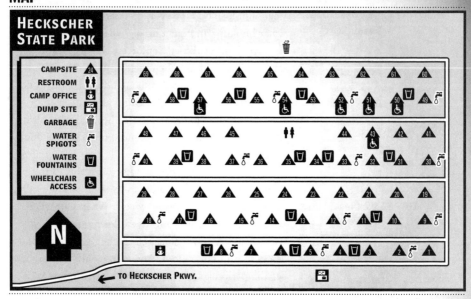

other area state parks during the length of their stay. Robert Moses State Park, at the western tip of Fire Island, is a popular nearby destination. Connected by a causeway, this is the only part of the Fire Island accessible by car, and it is home to the island's famous lighthouse.

Though the campground itself may not be particularly unique, Heckscher State Park is well worth a camping visit. New Yorkers find its proximity and the diversity of activities it offers particularly appealing. After all, it's the only park in the state where you can hike, bike, swim, sail, and see the New York Philharmonic perform every summer.

GETTING THERE

From Interstate 495, take Sagtikos Parkway South 4 miles to Southern State Parkway East (Heckscher Parkway). Take the Southern State Parkway East (Heckscher Parkway) 8 miles to the end. Park entrance is directly ahead.

GPS COORDINATES

PARK ENTRANCE:

UTM Zone (WGS84) 18T
Easting 655006
Northing 4508737
Latitude N 40°42'54"
Longitude W 73°09'53"

2
SEARS BELLOWS COUNTY PARK

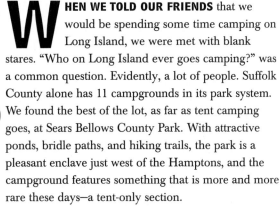

> *Pitch a tent in the calm, wooded surroundings of Long Island's pinelands.*

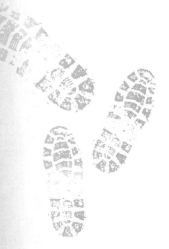

WHEN WE TOLD OUR FRIENDS that we would be spending some time camping on Long Island, we were met with blank stares. "Who on Long Island ever goes camping?" was a common question. Evidently, a lot of people. Suffolk County alone has 11 campgrounds in its park system. We found the best of the lot, as far as tent camping goes, at Sears Bellows County Park. With attractive ponds, bridle paths, and hiking trails, the park is a pleasant enclave just west of the Hamptons, and the campground features something that is more and more rare these days—a tent-only section.

To regulate use of its 48,000 acres of parkland, Suffolk County has instituted a system called the Green Key. Forget about trying to use your Empire Passport or ReserveAmerica. In Suffolk, the Green Key rules— and admittedly, the whole thing is a little complex. The Green Key is a pass (valid for three years) that county residents must purchase in order to receive reduced fees at county parks, as well as access to the golf course and campground-reservation system. Nonresidents can purchase a Tourist Green Key, which extends many of the same privileges, but it is more expensive and lasts only a year. Suffolk County residents probably already know all about this, but for more information on the byzantine rules explaining the procurement and use of the mighty key, call (631) 854-4949 or visit the Suffolk County Web site, **www.suffolkcountyny.gov.**

Once you have a Green Key, you're ready to start camping. And for tent campers, Sears Bellows is a good place to start. The park is not situated on the Atlantic or Long Island Sound, like most parks where RVs are the name of the game. It is inland, wedged at the bottleneck of land where the south fork of Long Island splits off. You can't play golf or water-ski here (or drink a beer for that matter), but you can pitch a

RATINGS

Beauty: ✿ ✿
Privacy: ✿ ✿
Quiet: ✿ ✿ ✿
Cleanliness: ✿ ✿
Security: ✿ ✿ ✿
Spaciousness: ✿ ✿ ✿

tent in the calm, wooded surroundings of Long Island's pinelands.

The campground's two loops are set off diagonally from each other and are split by the main park road. The trailer-only loop and group-camping sections are found just past the park office, to the right. Farther down the road and to the left is the tent-only section. There are 30 sites to choose from here, and all are relatively flat and surrounded by towering pines. If you are reserving a site online (which at the time of our research was only possible using Internet Explorer), the Web site informs you which have more shade. The exterior sites are generally more private, but the most isolated one we found was 23, an interior site.

Water spigots are well distributed, but if you're camping on the outer edge of the loop, you will have a short walk downhill to the comfort station. Overall, the accommodations are a bit rustic and, when we visited, could have used some more upkeep. Sites here are, however, a welcome change from the paved and cluttered ones you find elsewhere in the county. You feel as if you are in the thick of the woods here, even though the suburbs are not far away.

You can catch a glimpse of Bellows Pond from some of the sites, but none could be considered waterfront. Still, it's a quick hop down to the shores of Bellows, where you can go swimming at the beach from early June to Labor Day (when lifeguards are on duty) or grab a fishing pole, rent a rowboat, and try for some bluegill, bass, perch, and pickerel. There is a small activity field not far from the sites, but most people will want to spend more time at the beach or at the picnic pavilion and playground, both of which have great views. Reservations can be made for group events, and a large corner of the park across the water from the campground has been set off for this purpose. Many youth groups come here during the summer for camping, picnicking, and games.

Strap your boots and take off on some of the trails on dirt roads, and visit some of the park's other ponds. There are the three Munn's Ponds, along with Grass, Little House, Big House, and Division ponds, to say nothing of Sears Pond, the biggest of the bunch. The

KEY INFORMATION

ADDRESS:	Bellows Pond Road Hampton Bays, NY 11946
OPERATED BY:	Suffolk County Department of Parks, Recreation and Conservation
INFORMATION:	(631) 852-8290; www.suffolkcounty ny.gov
OPEN:	Early April–late May (Thursday–Saturday); late May–early September (all week)
SITES:	70 (30 tent-only, 40 trailer-only)
EACH SITE HAS:	Picnic table and fire ring
ASSIGNMENT:	Choose from available sites
REGISTRATION:	On arrival or by reservation
FACILITIES:	Water, flush toilets, showers, pay phone
PARKING:	At site, maximum 2 vehicles
FEE:	$14/night (Resident Green Key); $24/night (Tourist Key); $3/night reservation fee or $12 weekly reservation fee
ELEVATION:	20 feet
RESTRICTIONS:	*Pets:* Dogs on leash with proof of currently valid rabies vaccination, 2 pets maximum/site *Fires:* In fire rings only *Alcohol:* No alcohol permitted *Vehicles:* No limit *Other:* Quiet hours 10 p.m.–8 a.m. *Reservations:* 2- or 4-night stay required

MAP

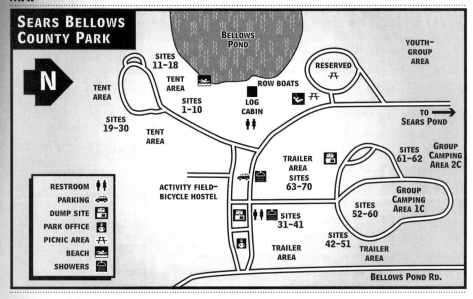

GETTING THERE

Follow NY 27 (Sunrise Highway) to Exit 65. Take NY 24 North and turn left on Bellows Pond Road. Park entrance is on your right.

GPS COORDINATES

PARK ENTRANCE:
UTM Zone (WGS84)   18T
Easting   706193
Northing   4529161
Latitude   N 40°53'15"
Longitude   W 72°33'09"

longest hiking trail, about 3 miles round-trip, leaves directly from the campground, crosses over bridle trails, and loops around shores of Sears. Speaking of bridle trails, they can be explored on horseback by shelling out a few dollars at the Sears Bellows Stables, which is on the northern edge of the park, right next to the Big Duck.

What is the Big Duck, you ask? Suffolk County calls it "Long Island's most famous landmark," and it is listed in the National Register of Historic Places. Basically, it's a gift shop and information booth in the shape of a giant white duck. Built in the 1930s, for many years it was a store that sold (what else?) ducks. In 1987, it was donated to the state, and since then it has served as a retailer of Long Island memorabilia (most of it duck themed) and a provider of tourist information. Hearing of this beloved monument, we imagined a towering roadside oddity and were a bit let down to see that it's smaller than some of today's RVs. But do stop by during your visit to Sears Bellows and learn a bit about the region. Chances are you will be surprised by the many outdoor adventures to be found in Suffolk County.

3
WATCH HILL

THERE ARE NO NATIONAL PARKS in New York state. However, just off the coast of Long Island is Fire Island National Seashore (operated by the National Park Service), a string of small communities connected by miles of undeveloped beach. And Watch Hill Campground, located on Fire Island, is where you'll find some of the best tent camping in the state. It is common in New York to find a campground near the beach. However, the landscape is spectacular at Watch Hill. With 26 walk-in sites situated among the dunes no more than 50 yards from the ocean, Watch Hill distinguishes itself as a campground that promises beach camping and actually delivers.

There are no roads running the length of Fire Island. Raised boardwalks above the dunes and marshes are the thoroughfares. Golf carts provide speedy travel for maintenance workers. Children's wagons serve as pack mules for groceries and supplies. No roads mean no cars and certainly no RVs. This makes getting to the island a little complicated, but it's worth the effort. From May through October, there is regular ferry service to Watch Hill from Patchogue, New York, with peak service (five to seven departures per day) during summer months. Be sure to call the Davis Park Ferry Company, (631) 475-1665, for an exact schedule, as it changes from month to month.

Upon reaching the island, the extensive marina grabs your attention. The park provides slips for visiting boaters, but don't worry about motor-related noise. The campground is still a quarter-mile away. At the marina you'll find the Watch Hill Visitor Center and Ranger Station, the dock shack (where campers check in), and a small store. When we visited, a snack bar was open, but the perennially popular dockside restaurant was under renovation and expected to open for the 2007 season.

> *At night, you will probably only hear the soft chatter of other campers, the gentle sounds of the wind and wildlife, and, on especially quiet evenings, the roar of the ocean.*

RATINGS

Beauty: ✿ ✿ ✿ ✿ ✿
Privacy: ✿ ✿ ✿ ✿
Quiet: ✿ ✿ ✿ ✿
Cleanliness: ✿ ✿ ✿ ✿
Security: ✿ ✿ ✿ ✿
Spaciousness: ✿ ✿ ✿

KEY INFORMATION

The campground is a five-minute walk from the marina, so a sturdy backpack to carry supplies would be useful. There are no ground fires allowed at sites, but each is equipped with a grill, and you'll definitely want to bring a bag of charcoal. You'll also want to load up on insect repellent and sunscreen. In the summer months, mosquitoes are thick; the sites are protected from the wind by shrubs, but there is little natural shade.

Boardwalks connect all the campground amenities, and buildings are raised to protect the dunes. The main boardwalk winds its way east from the marina to a comfort station with flush toilets and showers. One path continues south over the dunes to the beach. A narrower path leads east, directly to the camp- ground. The group, wheelchair-accessible, and host sites are the first you pass. The remaining sites are well distributed along the boardwalk, which is lined with fire extinguishers, water spigots, and one wash station.

When you arrive at Watch Hill, site selection is first come, first served. We recommend sites 2, 10, 25, and 26 for their privacy and distance from the board- walk. Campsites not directly connected to the board- walk can be accessed along sandy paths through other sites. The boardwalk through the camping area is popu- lar with day visitors, perhaps families exploring the area or local residents out jogging. At night, the only sounds you'll hear are the soft chatter of other campers, the gentle sounds of the wind and wildlife, and, on especially quiet evenings, the roar of the ocean.

Reservations are taken by mail only, starting on January 1 for the upcoming summer. Plan ahead, as spaces fill up by March for holidays and weekends. Application forms are available online or by calling the campground office. You will be able to choose from three possible visitation dates (in order of preference) and will be notified of your allotted date.

Although the campground is run by Fire Island Concessions, backcountry-camping permits are avail- able only through the National Park Service. There are many rules and regulations, and you will want to con- tact the Watch Hill Visitor Center for more details. Backcountry campers should be particularly careful about ticks and poison ivy.

MAP

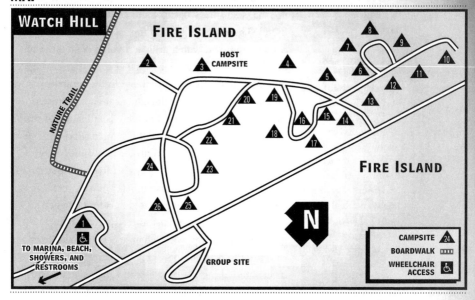

Spend some time exploring Davis Park, a charming community of seasonal homes a mile west of the campground. Closer in, a raised nature trail climbs through the narrow forest, providing great views of your tent before winding through the marshy northern side of the island. The Great South Bay spreads out before you, with the southern shore of Long Island, 4 miles away, usually visible. This loop trail showcases deer, rabbits, shorebirds, fish, and other local animals. Rangers conduct interpretive programs during the summer. A guided canoe trip is an enjoyable way to explore the area's salt marshes and tidal ecosystem.

The beach, understandably, is what attracts the most visitors. Follow the boardwalk to the beach to enjoy the sights, sounds, and smells of the Atlantic. Swimming is allowed only when lifeguards are present in summer. Watch for sections of beach roped off to protect the nesting areas of the federally protected piping plover. Be careful to stay off the dunes to preserve Fire Island for future visitors. Respecting this fragile barrier island will ensure it stays a summer destination for many generations.

GETTING THERE

From I-495, take Exit 63 to North Ocean Avenue (CR 83). Follow North Ocean Avenue south to Patchogue. Turn right onto Montauk Highway (NY 27A). Take the next left onto West Avenue. Drive one block. The parking lot for the Watch Hill Ferry Terminal is on the right.

GPS COORDINATES

WATCH HILL MARINA:

UTM Zone (WGS84)	18T
Easting	669816
Northing	4506545
Latitude	N 40°41'32"
Longitude	W 72°59'25"

4
WILDWOOD STATE PARK

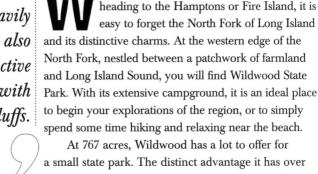

> *While it is heavily wooded, the park also contains an attractive beach bordered with steep, windswept bluffs.*

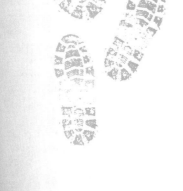

WHEN THE SUN COMES OUT and tourists are heading to the Hamptons or Fire Island, it is easy to forget the North Fork of Long Island and its distinctive charms. At the western edge of the North Fork, nestled between a patchwork of farmland and Long Island Sound, you will find Wildwood State Park. With its extensive campground, it is an ideal place to begin your explorations of the region, or to simply spend some time hiking and relaxing near the beach.

At 767 acres, Wildwood has a lot to offer for a small state park. The distinct advantage it has over most other parks is that it is heavily wooded and has an attractive beach bordered with steep, windswept bluffs. This combination keeps a steady stream of visitors, especially campers, coming and going throughout the summer months.

The park itself may be small, but the campground is the largest on Long Island. The 242 tent sites can fill quickly, so reservations are recommended on weekends and holidays. At other times, walk-ins should be easily accommodated.

When you enter the campground and register at the camp office, you will see a large RV camping area. Fortunately for tent campers, the park has separated these 80 electric-equipped sites from the more-remote tent sites. After registering, simply bear left from the office and follow the signs to the five tenting loops. You will first enter Loop B. In the spring and autumn months, only Loops B and D are open. After Memorial Day, all loops are open. Loops A and C are sandwiched in the middle of the campground. Loop E forms the far border and offers the most private camping experience.

All sites are wooded and well spaced. Naturally, sites along the outside edge of the loops are more secluded, but are also farthest from the comfort station. If you need a flat and dry surface on which to pitch

RATINGS

Beauty: ✿ ✿ ✿ ✿
Privacy: ✿ ✿ ✿
Quiet: ✿ ✿ ✿
Cleanliness: ✿ ✿ ✿ ✿
Security: ✿ ✿ ✿
Spaciousness: ✿ ✿ ✿ ✿

your tent, try Loop C. Equipped with wooden tent platforms—available for an extra $1 per night—Loop C is the most "civilized" of the loops. Some of the more spacious and private sites include C1, C19, D14, E24, and E25.

All sites lack both fire rings and grills. Fires are allowed, but only in approved containers with metal sides and bottoms. You can bring your own, but we recommend renting one from the campground vendor for $7.50 per night (with a $20 deposit). Quiet hours are from 10 p.m. to 7 a.m. Even though the RV section is removed from the tents, all campers will appreciate that generators are also prohibited during this time. Because of the campground's size, enforcing quiet hours isn't always the easiest task for the accommodating staff. But also because of its size, the campground is full of plenty of spots to find solitude.

Once you've established camp at Wildwood, take time to explore the North Fork of Long Island. Kids will probably beg to make a stop at Splish-Splash Water Park in Riverhead. The older crowd might find touring the many wineries that dot NY 25 more to their pace. Take the scenic drive out to Greenport to catch the ferry to Shelter Island, or continue on to Orient Beach State Park at the far eastern end of the fork.

If you choose to stay in the park, there is still plenty to do. During summer months, the campground offers movies, children's theater, square dancing, and magic and wildlife shows. A bike rally and a fall festival are annual events.

Color-coded hiking and biking trails, including an 11-mile loop, circle the park. Nearly three-fourths of the land is undeveloped hardwood forest. Exploring these trails is a great way to enjoy some quiet time away from the campground. One of the most popular hikes starts where the Pedestrian Walk meets the beach parking lot. The trail meanders for nearly 4 miles, opening onto the bluffs and lovely views of Long Island Sound.

The beach itself is a short stroll from the campground along the Pedestrian Walk, but some campers choose to drive to the closer visitor lot. A large picnic area, playground, and concession stands surround the

KEY INFORMATION

ADDRESS:	P.O. Box 518 Hulse Landing Road Wading River, NY 11792
OPERATED BY:	New York State Office of Parks, Recreation and Historic Preservation
INFORMATION:	(631) 929-4314; nysparks.state .ny.us
OPEN:	Early April–early October
SITES:	322 (80 electrical hookups)
EACH SITE HAS:	Picnic table
ASSIGNMENT:	Choose from available sites or reservations
REGISTRATION:	On arrival
FACILITIES:	Water, flush toilets, showers, dump station, camp store, pay phone
PARKING:	At site, 1 vehicle maximum, 1 additional car at separate lot for fee
FEE:	$14/night (plus $3/night on Friday, Saturday, and holidays)
ELEVATION:	167 feet
RESTRICTIONS:	*Pets:* Not allowed *Fires:* In approved containers only (available for rent at campground office) *Alcohol:* Prohibited *Vehicles:* Up to 50 feet *Other:* Quiet hours 10 p.m.–7 a.m. *Reservations:* 2-night stay required

MAP

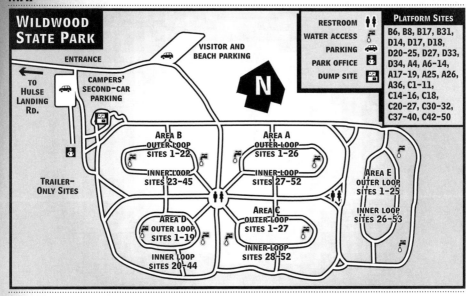

GETTING THERE

From I-495, take Exit 68 to NY 46 North. Follow NY 46 North for 7 miles to NY 25A East. Bear right onto Sound Avenue. Turn left at traffic light onto Hulse Landing Road. Park entrance is on the right.

GPS COORDINATES

PARK ENTRANCE:
UTM Zone (WGS84)   18T
Easting   684352
Northing   4536916
Latitude   N 40°57'45"
Longitude   W 72°48'33"

lot, shaded throughout by tall trees. During the summer, this day-use area attracts many local visitors, who pack up the family and walk down the steep, paved path to the beach.

A bathhouse (with another concession stand) sits squarely in the center of the beach, but the main draw is the water and the beauty of the bluffs. The high, sandy bluffs slope down to a narrow beach and rolling waves. Because of erosion, the bluffs, with their delicate vegetation, are strictly off-limits. The beach stretches far in both directions, with fishing and bathing areas clearly designated. But if you just want to take it easy, sitting in the sand and looking out onto the Long Island Sound is an appealing option.

The combination of forest and beach attracts visitors for numerous reasons. According to one campground worker, "lots of city folks" come out each summer. But the campground appeals to many people, including that same employee, who told us that he planned to spend his vacation time camping with friends at Wildwood.

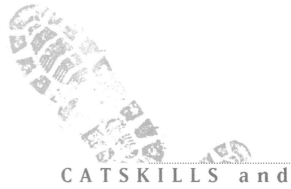

CATSKILLS and
HUDSON VALLEY

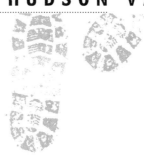

5
CLARENCE FAHNESTOCK MEMORIAL STATE PARK

FOR THE **88** MILES IT PASSES through New York state, the Appalachian Trail meanders over relatively flat, wooded terrain, never rising past 1,500 feet. For some, it is one of the least memorable sections of the trail. More than 10 miles of the route, however, passes through Clarence Fahnestock Memorial State Park, a 12,000-acre gem with some of the best hiking in the Hudson Highlands. And just a few hundred yards from the famed trail is an attractive campground, nestled into one of the park's many ridges.

Along the scenic Taconic State Parkway and only 60 miles from New York City, Fahnestock, as it is commonly called, attracts plenty of visitors looking for short day hikes. There are plenty of brief rambles to be experienced, but the tent camper will discover that the park deserves at least a few days of exploration. Not only does it serve as a jumping off (or stopping off) point for the Appalachian Trail, it also features seven small mountains to summit, a series of attractive lakes and ponds, horse and bike paths, and a good-sized beach for summertime swimming.

For us, the campground itself was worth the visit. While many campgrounds are no more than wooded parking lots, the one at Fahnestock is distinguished by roads that twist around large seams of stone jutting up among the trees. Tucked into the rock outcroppings, the sites offer more isolation from neighbors than one might expect and are relatively flat compared to the rolling roads. The first section (1 through 29) includes a series of walk-in sites set about 30 yards from the road. It is a short distance, but with all the cars for these sites parked along the camp road, it can at least give the illusion that you are "packing it in."

Sites 25 and 30, perched up among the rocks and well shaded, are among the most desirable. The most spacious sites, numbered 30 through 50, are those spread out on the loop near Pelton Pond. Further along

> *Fahnestock is distinguished by roads that twist around large seams of stone jutting up among the trees.*

RATINGS

Beauty: ✿ ✿ ✿ ✿
Privacy: ✿ ✿ ✿ ✿
Quiet: ✿ ✿ ✿ ✿
Cleanliness: ✿ ✿
Security: ✿ ✿ ✿
Spaciousness: ✿ ✿ ✿ ✿

ADDRESS: 1498 Route 301
Carmel, NY 10512

OPERATED BY: New York State
Office of Parks,
Recreation and His-
toric Preservation

INFORMATION: 845-225-7207;
nysparks.state.ny.us

OPEN: Late April–early
December

SITES: 80

EACH SITE HAS: Picnic table, grill,
and fire ring

ASSIGNMENT: Choose from
available sites or
reservations

REGISTRATION: On arrival

FACILITIES: Water, pit and flush
toilets, showers, pay
phone, laundry

PARKING: At site, maximum
2 vehicles

FEE: $13/night (plus
$3/night for
Friday, Saturday,
and holidays)

ELEVATION: 1,059 feet

RESTRICTIONS: *Pets:* Dogs in campsites 70–81 on leash
with proof of cur-
rently valid rabies
vaccination
Fires: In fire rings or
grills only
Alcohol: At site
Vehicles: Up to 30 feet
Other: Quiet hours
10 p.m.–7 a.m.;
Swimming only in
Canopus Lake when
lifeguard present
(weekends in June,
daily in July and
August); no gas
motors in Canopus
Lake; no swimming
or boats in Pelton
Pond
Reservations: 2-night
stay required

the road are three grassy lots that essentially serve as sites 51 through 81. The only good reason to stay in these crowded sections is if you bring a pet, as dogs are only allowed at sites 70 through 81. Two comfort stations serve opposite ends of the campground. Though all sites are technically for tents or trailers, tents prevail throughout Fahnestock. There are no hookups or dumping station for RVs.

Pelton Pond, a small body of water at the edge of the campground, is great spot to cast a fishing line. Neither swimming nor boating is allowed, but the pond is regularly stocked with rainbow trout. Nearby John Allen Pond and Canopus Lake are also chock-full of bass, perch, and sunfish. Anglers must obtain a New York state fishing license before cracking open their tackle boxes. And those wishing to fish the park's Stillwater Lake must obtain an additional permit from the park office.

The park's Taconic Education Center is mainly for reserved group use, but the nature center at the northern point of Pelton Pond offers interpretive programs on summer weekends. The 1.5-mile Pelton Pond Nature Trail is a nice little loop that will introduce visitors to the flora and fauna of the area. But the white blazes of the Appalachian Trail are what will draw a large number of hikers. A 5-mile segment of the trail can be followed from the south end of Canopus Lake up along a ridge to great views of the area. One of the park's brochures recommends doing the hike in June, when the mountain laurels are in bloom. There are more than 42 miles of trails to choose from in the park.

Anglers will want to take the 6-mile Three Lakes Hike, which showcases the three larger fishing spots mentioned above and follows a former mine-railroad path. The region was mined for iron ore for nearly 100 years, ending in 1876, when competition got the best of the local industry. A Manhattan doctor named Clarence Fahnestock purchased sections of what is now the park in the early 20th century. He died during World War I in France, and his family donated the land to the state for the creation of the park in his memory.

After a day of hiking, the spring-fed Canopus Lake and its large, man-made beach offer a refreshing respite. The soft white sand attracts many bathers and

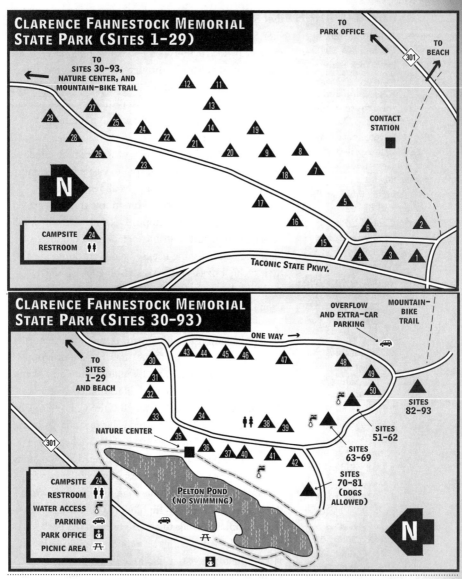

CLARENCE FAHNESTOCK MEMORIAL STATE PARK (SITES 1–29)

TO PARK OFFICE

TO BEACH

301

TO SITES 30–93, NATURE CENTER, AND MOUNTAIN–BIKE TRAIL

CONTACT STATION

N

CAMPSITE 24
RESTROOM

TACONIC STATE PKWY.

CLARENCE FAHNESTOCK MEMORIAL STATE PARK (SITES 30–93)

OVERFLOW AND EXTRA-CAR PARKING

MOUNTAIN–BIKE TRAIL

ONE WAY

TO SITES 1–29 AND BEACH

301

NATURE CENTER

SITES 82–93

SITES 51–62

SITES 63–69

SITES 70–81 (DOGS ALLOWED)

PELTON POND (NO SWIMMING)

CAMPSITE 24
RESTROOM
WATER ACCESS
PARKING
PARK OFFICE
PICNIC AREA

N

is extremely popular for day-use visitors; campers enjoy free access and may bring two cars to the parking lot. This beach offers a concession stand, showers, grills, swimming, boat rentals, and more—certainly enough to keep campers busy and cool on a hot summer day. Be sure to enjoy a cold swim and the nice thought that you're sleeping just across the road.

GETTING THERE

From Taconic State Parkway, take CR 301 West for 0.25 miles to park entrances.

GPS COORDINATES

UTM Zone (WGS84)	18T
Easting	598124
Northing	4591124
Latitude	N 41°27'57"
Longitude	W 73°49'30"

6
DEVIL'S TOMBSTONE

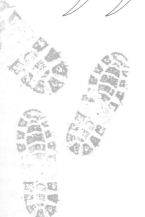

> *Some claim the satanic nomenclature is still appropriate today, as this is the jumping-off point for one of the most challenging hikes in the Catskills, the Devil's Path Trail.*

TRADITIONAL **D**UTCH GHOST STORIES often tell of the Devil's presence in Stony Clove, a pass through the Devil's Path Range. Today, Stony Clove is better known as County Route 214, connecting the modern-day towns of Phoenecia and Hunter. The pass may be paved over, but the boulder known as the Devil's Tombstone remains. Almost seven feet high and five feet across, the impressive monolith can be found at the southern end of the humble campground that bears its name. It has been there for as long as anyone knows.

Surrounded by the Indian Head Wilderness, Devil's Tombstone is a secluded, primitive campground, only 4 miles from town, but seemingly far removed from civilization. It is one of the oldest collections of sites in the state, and CR 214 is the main reminder of the modern world. The road runs through the middle of the campground, dividing it into two sections of equal size. During the day, cars can be both seen and heard from most sites. Once the sun sets, traffic reduces to a trickle, and it is unlikely you will even remember the road is there.

Upon arrival, be prepared to spend a little time checking in. Crowds are scarce and you probably won't be waiting in any lines, but the campground office is powered by a generator, which hardly provides enough energy to run the computer and printer at the same time. The ranger may treat you to tales of woebegone campers ignorant of how to pitch a tent, let alone start a fire, as he plugs your information into the database by the light of gas lamps.

They call Devil's Tombstone primitive camping, but the primary difference between this and other campgrounds in the region is the lack of running water in the comfort stations and the carry-out policy for all trash. The pit toilets are well maintained, and the comfort

RATINGS

Beauty: ✿ ✿ ✿
Privacy: ✿ ✿ ✿
Quiet: ✿ ✿ ✿ ✿
Cleanliness: ✿ ✿ ✿ ✿
Security: ✿ ✿
Spaciousness: ✿ ✿ ✿

stations are even decorated with garlands of silk flowers. Potable-water spigots are well distributed throughout the campground. Supplies and groceries can be obtained in Hunter, a popular resort town only a few miles to the north. Campers in desperate need of a hot shower or a dip in a cold lake can drive a few miles east to Tannersville and use their Devil's Tombstone registration to gain free access to the facilities at North-South Lake (profiled later in this chapter).

The sites themselves are ample enough, and unless you're visiting on a holiday, it's rare to find the campground at capacity. On weekdays, only four or five sites at most may be filled. Personally, we found sites 3 and 4 on the eastern half of the campground the most desirable for their privacy. Some people prefer the western end, however, because it borders on Stony Clove Creek. Whether the creek is actually flowing when you visit is another story. Fed by the overflow of nearby Notch Lake, it will often run dry when rain hasn't made a recent visit. Partly because of the lack of facilities and possibly due to the challenging nature of the nearby hiking, the campground attracts fewer families and many more backpackers and young couples.

Some claim the satanic nomenclature is still appropriate today, as this is the jumping-off point for one of the most challenging hikes in the Catskills, the steep, rugged Devil's Path Trail. Just past the north end of the campground is a small parking lot bordering Notch Lake. At this point, the Devil's Path Trail bisects the road, leading west to limited views, including a fire tower. To the east is the Plateau Hike, one of the most popular choices for day visitors because it provides gorgeous views of so many mountains that it is unclear where one ends and the next begins. The Plateau Hike takes about two hours round-trip, but this is hardly an afternoon ramble. The stony trail rises 1,700 feet in only 1.5 miles, ascending through dense forest. From the top, there are views of Hunter Mountain across Stony Clove, and Slide Mountain rises to the south. The trail then loops around, offering views of Roundtop and Kaaterskill High Peak to the east. The Hudson Valley— and even Stratton and Mount Snow in Vermont—can be seen on clear days. Following the trail east will test

KEY INFORMATION

ADDRESS:	County Route 214 P.O. Box 6 Hunter, NY 12442
OPERATED BY:	New York State Department of Environmental Conservation
INFORMATION:	(845) 688-7160; www.dec.state.ny .us/website/do/ camping
OPEN:	Mid-May–early September
SITES:	24
EACH SITE HAS:	Picnic table and fire ring
ASSIGNMENT:	Choose from available sites or reservations
REGISTRATION:	On arrival
FACILITIES:	Water, pit toilets, pay phone
PARKING:	At site, maximum 2 vehicles
FEE:	$12/night
ELEVATION:	1,902 feet
RESTRICTIONS:	*Pets:* Dogs on leash with proof of currently valid rabies vaccination *Fires:* In fire rings only *Alcohol:* At site *Vehicles:* Up to 30 feet *Other:* Quiet hours 10 p.m.–7 a.m.; no swimming or boating; carry out all trash *Reservations:* 2-night stay required

MAP

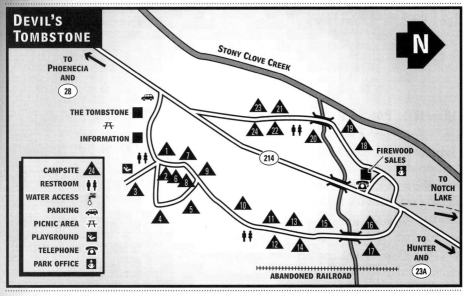

DEVIL'S TOMBSTONE

TO PHOENECIA AND **28**

THE TOMBSTONE

INFORMATION

CAMPSITE	▲24
RESTROOM	👫
WATER ACCESS	💧
PARKING	🚗
PICNIC AREA	🎋
PLAYGROUND	🛝
TELEPHONE	☎
PARK OFFICE	🚹

STONY CLOVE CREEK

214

FIREWOOD SALES

TO NOTCH LAKE

TO HUNTER AND **23A**

ABANDONED RAILROAD

N

GETTING THERE

From Interstate 87 (New York State Thruway), take Exit 19, Kingston, to NY 28 West. Follow NY 28 to Phoenecia. In the town of Phoenecia, follow signs for CR 214. Drive 9 miles; the campground entrance is on the left.

even the most seasoned backpackers, but will reward those that do with an authentic experience of the Indian Head Wilderness.

It would be difficult to overestimate the importance of this wild region. The Tombstone itself expresses this quite clearly. It holds a plaque from 1985 commemorating the 100th anniversary of New York's Forest Preserve, ending with the words, "The surrounding mountains, streams and woodlands remain a legacy from the past protected by the constitution of New York State. They represent a heritage for future generations."

GPS COORDINATES

PARK ENTRANCE:

UTM Zone (WGS84) 18T
Easting 565437
Northing 4666936
Latitude N 42°09'07"
Longitude W 74°12'29"

7
LITTLE POND

Andes

LITTLE POND CAMPGROUND perches on the western edge of the Catskill Forest Preserve, just south of the Delaware River. Perhaps more than any other campground in the region, Little Pond offers the solitude of wilderness camping with the amenities of a well-run facility.

Don't let the word *pond* (or *little*, for that matter) fool you. In New York's Catskill and Adirondack mountains, many bodies of water are dubbed ponds that in different settings would qualify as lakes. At 13 acres, Little Pond may not hold a candle to one of the Great Lakes, but it is hardly a puddle. Forested on all sides (and with no motorboats allowed), it is a quiet spot to fish, swim, or paddle around in a small boat. And with a campground tucked along the southern shores, Little Pond makes for an excellent weekend getaway.

What struck us most about Little Pond Campground when we first entered was how lush the surroundings were. They bring to mind the Great Smoky Mountains in June. The area is thin on population, but thick with wildlife. Upon registering, visitors are asked to read and sign a "Bear Warning and Guidelines Notification," outlining precautions to take when camping in the vicinity of black bears. New York has a population of approximately 7,000 black bears, and the region around Little Pond is indeed bear country. Although sightings are rare, for your own (as well as the bears') safety, you should take the guidelines seriously. It is easy to forget how dangerous bears can be. As one local ranger told us, "If you feed the chipmunks, you eventually feed the bears."

The main camping area is divided into two sections, separated by a stream and a small pool of muddy water, which is perhaps more befitting of the campground's name. The loops are wooded, with tall trees rising from the red dirt. Rolling hills increase

> *Perhaps more than any other campground in the region, Little Pond offers the solitude of wilderness camping with the amenities of a well-run facility.*

RATINGS

Beauty: ✿ ✿ ✿ ✿
Privacy: ✿ ✿ ✿ ✿
Quiet: ✿ ✿ ✿ ✿
Cleanliness: ✿ ✿ ✿
Security: ✿ ✿ ✿
Spaciousness: ✿ ✿ ✿ ✿

ADDRESS:	Barkaboom Road Andes, NY 13731
OPERATED BY:	New York State Department of Environmental Conservation
INFORMATION:	(845) 439-5480; www.dec.state.ny.us/ website/do/camping
OPEN:	Mid-May– mid-October
SITES:	75 (including 8 walk-in sites)
EACH SITE HAS:	Picnic table and fire ring
ASSIGNMENT:	Choose from available sites or reservations
REGISTRATION:	On arrival
FACILITIES:	Water, pit and flush toilets, showers, pay phone
PARKING:	At site, maximum 2 vehicles or designated lot for walk-in sites
FEE:	$18/night
ELEVATION:	1,657 feet
RESTRICTIONS:	*Pets:* Dogs on leash with proof of currently valid rabies vaccination *Fires:* In fire rings only *Alcohol:* At site *Vehicles:* No maximum *Other:* Quiet hours 10 p.m.–7 a.m.; no motorized boats in Little Pond *Reservations:* 2-night stay required

the sense of privacy. Each campsite features a fire ring, a picnic table, and a nice flat place for a tent. Sites 1 through 20 are less hilly, a little more open, and farther from Little Pond. Sites 7, 8, 61, and 62 have views of the stream and the muddy pool. Some of the more popular sites are 25, 26, 35, 36, and 37, coveted for their proximity to Little Pond.

In addition to the main camping area, eight remote (i.e. walk-in) sites are scattered along the north end of Little Pond. The parking lot for campers staying at these sites also serves the pond's small boat ramp. A gravel nature trail with sturdy wooden bridges across streams starts at the lot and passes by an old stone fireplace before reaching the first site about 100 yards farther along. The sites are designated from 68 to 75, each with its own pit toilet and a view of the water. Site 71 is the most removed from the trail and closest to water. Site 73 offers excellent views. You may want to forgo site 72. Jutted up against the trail and small, it's the least appealing option. Follow the trail past site 75 and skirt the edge of the pond until you soon reach the day-use area. This short Loop Trail, as it is known, is enjoyed by many families during the day, but when the sun goes down, the walk-in sites are quiet and private—a treat for tent campers.

Fishing is popular in Little Pond, whether from the grassy banks, off the fishing pier, or over the edge of a boat. Canoes, kayaks, and rowboats are all available to rent, either by the hour or the day. Just down the road, the Beaverkill and the East Branch of the Delaware River are popular with fly fishers. The largest bodies of water in the Catskills are a series of reservoirs that supply New York City. The nearby Pepacton Reservoir is full of large trout and bass, but permits obtained from New York City are needed to fish it.

If you're not an angler, you might enjoy the swimming beach, picnic area, and hot showers. In the summer, the campground offers a junior naturalist program for kids of all ages. Stock up on supplies at the Turnwood General Store less than a mile from the campground entrance. And if the nature trail is too short a jaunt for your tastes, you can set out from the day-use area and explore the base of Touchmenot Mountain and

MAP

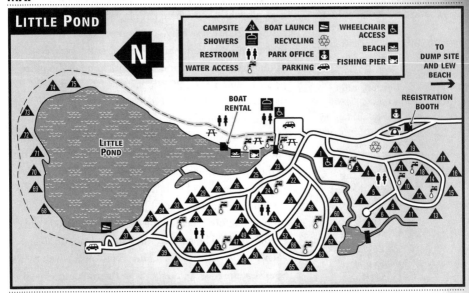

trails that continue on for miles to the east and west. Chances are, many folks will choose simply to stay at their campsites and enjoy the quiet surroundings.

GETTING THERE

From NY 17, take Exit 96, Livingston Manor, to Old Route 17. Follow Old Route 17 for 1 mile and turn right onto CR 151. Follow CR 151 through the town of Lew Beach. Approximately 10 miles from Lew Beach make a left on Big Pond Road. Drive an eighth of a mile to the campground entrance on the left.

GPS COORDINATES

PARK ENTRANCE:

UTM Zone (WGS84)	18T
Easting	522544
Northing	4653770
Latitude	N 42°02'08"
Longitude	W 74°43'39"

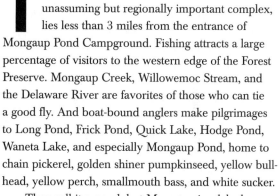

8
MONGAUP POND

> *Gas engines are prohibited, making for a calm, leisurely spirit on the water.*

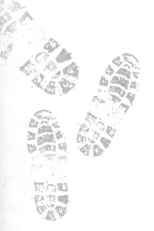

THE **CATSKILL FISH HATCHERY,** a rather unassuming but regionally important complex, lies less than 3 miles from the entrance of Mongaup Pond Campground. Fishing attracts a large percentage of visitors to the western edge of the Forest Preserve. Mongaup Creek, Willowemoc Stream, and the Delaware River are favorites of those who can tie a good fly. And boat-bound anglers make pilgrimages to Long Pond, Frick Pond, Quick Lake, Hodge Pond, Waneta Lake, and especially Mongaup Pond, home to chain pickerel, golden shiner pumpkinseed, yellow bullhead, yellow perch, smallmouth bass, and white sucker.

They call it a pond, but Mongaup is a lake by most standards, and at 122 acres, it is actually the largest body of water in the Catskills outside of the reservoirs that serve New York City. Gas engines are prohibited, making for a calm, leisurely spirit on the water. The car-top boat launch next to the fishing pier sees a lot of traffic, and rowboats and canoes are plentiful (and available for rent). At the southern end of the pond are a lifeguard station and a roped-off section of water for swimming. The large sandy beach, picnic area, and volleyball net draw some day-use visitors in addition to campers.

During the summer, organized environmental and recreational activities for both children and adults are posted in the *Wilderness Times,* a newsletter available at the ranger station. The campground also participates in the state-run Junior Naturalist Program. Children between the ages of 5 and 12 can fill out a wildlife journal to earn a colorful patch. A recent year's patch depicted a black bear, which are actually somewhat common in surrounding Sullivan County. The staff asks campers registering to sign a bear-notification form and warns them to take precautions, including not sleeping in clothes worn while cooking.

RATINGS

Beauty: ✿ ✿ ✿
Privacy: ✿ ✿ ✿
Quiet: ✿ ✿ ✿ ✿
Cleanliness: ✿ ✿ ✿ ✿
Security: ✿ ✿ ✿ ✿
Spaciousness: ✿ ✿ ✿ ✿ ✿

Isolation reigns at Mongaup, and there is no private development on the lake—just the seven loops of sites, all suitable for tents or RVs. The sections are so well spaced that it is easy to forget there are more than 160 sites. Each is standard-issue, but a few small touches in the campground really stand out. The faux stone on fireplaces and bright flowers planted by the showers and boat ramp are evidence of a well-maintained facility. The occasional pop-up will stop over for a visit, but even fewer RVs pass through the gates. Families in tents are definitely the majority here. The staff is very conscious of human impact on the campground and encourages campers to stay in the middle of their sites to prevent them from expanding over time.

Loops A, B, and C are spread out along the southeast section of the pond, just past the registration booth. In general, the interior sections of the loops provide less privacy but are closer to the comfort stations. Loops A and B are not on the lake and include some of the more crowded sites, such as 32 through 36, 53, 55, and 67 through 69. Behind sites 42, 44, and 46, a large field calls out for a game of ball. Loop C has a smattering of sites with water views, but the more spacious Loops D, E, F, and G offer better options for those seeking memorable views. Loops D and E contain the largest sites available, sitting beneath the shade of older hardwoods. On Loops F and G, denser, smaller trees and shrubs envelop the sites, and campers are guaranteed a little more privacy. The waterfront sites at Loop F are some of the most popular, most notably 122 through 124, 126 through 130, and 132 through 136. Loop G, the farthest from both the registration booth and day-use area, is also not too shabby. For a quieter waterfront sojourn, 139 through 144 are the best options.

The twisting coastline of Mongaup Pond allows for a total of 50 sites with water views. But few are directly at the water's edge. That's not such a bad thing, for it increases the sense of seclusion when looking out over the pond. But at night, it's certainly pleasant to see the twinkling lights of campfires across the water.

Supplies are easy to come by, as the "Woodman" and "Happy Trails" traveling stores, in the form of pickup trucks or small vans, circle the loops at least

THE BEST IN TENT CAMPING NEW YORK STATE

MAP

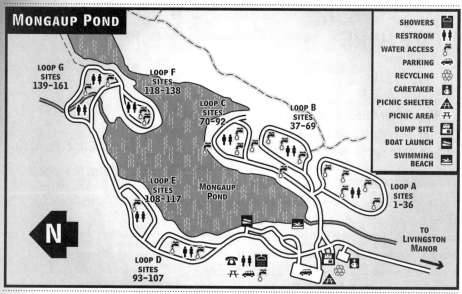

MONGAUP POND

LOOP G
SITES
139-161

LOOP F
SITES
118-138

LOOP C
SITES
70-92

LOOP B
SITES
37-69

LOOP E
SITES
108-117

MONGAUP
POND

LOOP A
SITES
1-36

LOOP D
SITES
93-107

N

TO
LIVINGSTON
MANOR

SHOWERS
RESTROOM
WATER ACCESS
PARKING
RECYCLING
CARETAKER
PICNIC SHELTER
PICNIC AREA
DUMP SITE
BOAT LAUNCH
SWIMMING
BEACH

GETTING THERE

From NY 17, take Exit 96,
Livingston Manor, to CR
81/82 for 6 miles. In the village of Debruce, turn left
on Mongaup Road/Fish
Hatchery Road. Follow Mongaup Road/Fish Hatchery
Road 3 miles to campground
entrance straight ahead.

GPS COORDINATES

PARK ENTRANCE:

UTM Zone (WGS84) 18T
Easting   525574
Northing   4644974
Latitude   N 41°57'23"
Longitude W 74°41'29"

once every evening. In addition to helping keep you
or your food warm, the Woodman sells ice to keep your
drinks and perishables cool. Happy Trails provides
everything campers could need, ranging from food
(ice cream, chips, soda) to practical (duct tape, batteries,
bug spray) and purely fun items (magic-grow capsules,
glow sticks, hula hoops).

For those seeking activities beyond their sites,
there are miles of multiuse trails nearby. A popular
short hike is the 3.5-mile Waterfall Loop, which passes
a cascade of water and the site of an old sawmill.
Hikers will find trails to Long Pond and Mongaup
Mountain leaving directly from the campground. The
Frick Pond trailhead, offering longer trails to the northwest, has its own parking lot, located down a short
road to the west just before the campground entrance.

Whether you are looking for boating, swimming,
hiking, or just a nice campfire, Mongaup Pond is sure
to offer something for all tent campers. Be sure to pull
out that tackle box, though. About 58 tons of brown
trout are produced at the hatchery every year and
released locally. You're bound to pull up a pound or
two in nearby waters.

9 MILLS-NORRIE STATE PARK

OGDEN MILLS AND RUTH LIVINGSTON MILLS Memorial State Park borders and shares a campground with Margaret Lewis Norrie State Park. The campground is technically located in Margaret Lewis Norrie, but understandably, its name was shortened to Mills-Norrie. Both parks are on the banks of the Hudson River, and this is the state-park campground that's closest to the river. The Norrie Marina, which consists of a large boat launch and 145 rental slips, serves the campground and makes getting onto the water a snap.

We are unhappy to report that the campground is not directly on the water. It is perched upon a densely wooded hill, and the trees are too thick and the topography too sloped to afford river views. Unless you reserve one of the parks' ten rental cabins, you will not be greeted by New York's most famous river when you wake. This is a blessing in some ways. Water views bring the unrelenting hordes, and Mills-Norrie is thankfully far from crowded.

This is one of the few state-park campgrounds without a registration booth. When you arrive, signs instruct you to find your reserved site, set up camp, and wait for park staff to register you. If you don't have reservations, that doesn't seem to be a problem, either. Just find a vacant site, pitch your tent, and, again, wait for registration. This policy may change if the campground becomes more popular, but for now it's a welcome alternative to waiting at a campground gate while park staff struggles with slow computers.

Another welcome surprise at Mills-Norrie is the lack of RVs. There were none there when we visited, and only a handful of pop-ups. RVs are certainly allowed and a few will make an appearance, but the sites themselves are small and somewhat crowded— a shame as far as privacy is concerned, but an obvious

> *This is where history and nature meet.*

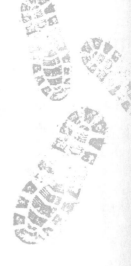

RATINGS

Beauty: ✿ ✿
Privacy: ✿ ✿
Quiet: ✿ ✿ ✿
Cleanliness: ✿ ✿
Security: ✿ ✿
Spaciousness: ✿ ✿

ADDRESS: Old Post Road, P.O. Box 893 Staatsburg, NY 12580

OPERATED BY: New York State Office of Parks, Recreation and Historic Preservation

INFORMATION: (845) 889-4646; nysparks.state.ny.us

OPEN: Mid-May– late October

SITES: 46

EACH SITE HAS: Picnic table and fire ring

ASSIGNMENT: Choose from available sites or reservations

REGISTRATION: On arrival

FACILITIES: Water, flush toilets, hot showers, pay phone

PARKING: At site, maximum 2 vehicles

FEE: $13/night (plus $3/night on Friday, Saturday, and holidays)

ELEVATION: 30 feet

RESTRICTIONS: *Pets:* Dogs on leash with proof of currently valid rabies vaccination
Fires: In fire rings only
Alcohol: At site
Vehicles: Up to 40 feet
Other: Quiet hours 10 p.m.–7 a.m.
Reservations: 2-night stay required

deterrent to noisy behemoths. The short, rough, intersecting roads may also help keep some trailers away.

The sites are arranged in a single loop, and as with many other campgrounds, the nicest spaces are located on the outer edge. Sites 48 and 49 are among the most private. Site 44, along the eastern edge, is not a bad option, but it's a bit exposed. The most coveted site would have to be 10. In the northeast corner, it is isolated, and if you walk a few paces and strain your eyes a bit, you might actually see the Hudson. In general, the campground fills up only on holiday weekends, so you can either reserve a site along the edge or simply show up and see which one strikes your fancy.

What brings most people to the campground is the chance to get their boat onto the Hudson. While you can't launch your boat from your site, you are allowed to store it there, so long as it fits. Many locals rent seasonal slips at the bustling Norrie Marina, which is just down the road but well separated from the campground. No swimming is allowed in the park, so most campers use the marina to launch small vessels, including plenty of kayaks. Campers often leave cars and boat trailers in the marina's parking lot. An environmental center, just south of the lot at the very edge of the park boundary, offers programs here on Saturdays in the summer. It is also a good place to set off on some of parks' trails and into almost 1,000 acres of forests and fields.

For gorgeous vistas of the Hudson, grab the trail map from the environmental center and take a hike north on the White Trail, which visits the campground and follows along bluffs, high above the water. The Horse Trail and the Mills Historic Trail make their way through the center of the parks, the latter ending at Mills Mansion, a pillared 79-room Beaux Arts estate donated by the Mills family to the state in 1938. Tours are available Wednesdays through Sundays during camping season. For a short, looping stroll, try the Yellow Trail, which can be accessed from a parking lot near the campground. Three other color-blazed trails— Blue, Red, and Green—follow old dirt roads, and double as cross-country ski paths in the winter.

Mills-Norrie is truly at the heart of the historic Hudson Valley, where industrialists and influential

MAP

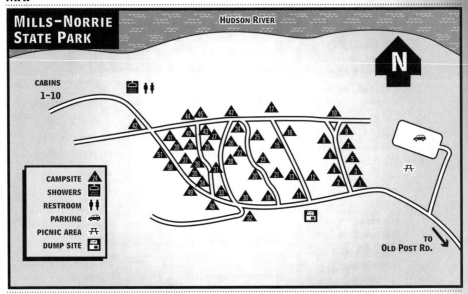

figures maintained extravagant homes. Aside from Mills Mansion, many other important buildings are minutes away. Five miles south is the town of Hyde Park, home to the Vanderbilt Mansion, Franklin Delano Roosevelt's Springwood and Presidential Library, and Eleanor Roosevelt's cottage, Val-Kill. Hop over the Mid-Hudson Bridge and drive about 40 minutes to visit Mohonk Mountain House, an elegant and gigantic castle that is one the country's most famous hotels. You won't have to book a room, but you will have to pay an entrance fee to explore the estate's impeccable gardens and miles of hiking trails.

Admittedly, the campground at Mills-Norrie is not the most inspired. It could use some more maintenance (though the comfort stations were clean and new), and security is not its strong point. It is, however, in a wonderful location, close to the wide shores of the Hudson. More than anywhere else in the state, this is where history and nature meet. Whether by boat, by foot, or by car, you can easily access it all from Mills-Norrie.

GETTING THERE

From I-87 (New York State Thruway), take Exit 19, Kingston. Follow NY 199 East over the Kingston-Rhinecliff Bridge to US 9G South. Follow US 9G South for 1.5 miles, then turn right on US 9 South. Follow US 9 South to village of Staatsburg; turn right on Old Post Road. Park entrance is on right.

GPS COORDINATES

PARK ENTRANCE:
UTM Zone (WGS84)   18T
Easting   588798
Northing   4632595
Latitude   N 41°50'25"
Longitude   W 73°55'50"

10
NORTH–SOUTH
LAKE

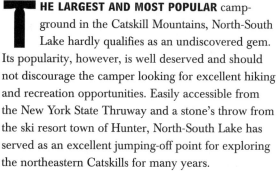

> *For a community-camping experience, North-South Lake is fantastic during the summer.*

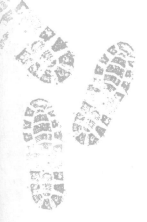

THE LARGEST AND MOST POPULAR camp-ground in the Catskill Mountains, North-South Lake hardly qualifies as an undiscovered gem. Its popularity, however, is well deserved and should not discourage the camper looking for excellent hiking and recreation opportunities. Easily accessible from the New York State Thruway and a stone's throw from the ski resort town of Hunter, North-South Lake has served as an excellent jumping-off point for exploring the northeastern Catskills for many years.

Even those who have never visited the area may recognize the scenery from the work of the Hudson River School of early American painters. Nearby Kaaterskill Falls, the highest falls in the state, is depicted in Thomas Cole's *Falls of the Katerskill* [sic], and North-South Lake served as inspiration to Jasper Francis Cropsey and his 1850 painting *Catskill Creek.*

The name "North-South Lake" is in itself curious. It is currently a single lake, but for most of its history, an earthen dam in a narrow isthmus separated the lake into two bodies of water. A state-run campground was first established on North Lake in 1929, consisting of just ten sites. Yet it was not until 1984, when the state purchased South Lake from a private owner, that the dam was removed and North-South Lake in its present form was born. People still refer to North Lake *and* South Lake for the sake of clarity.

While the number of campsites in the campground has blossomed to 219 over the years, the sites are still restricted to the shores and surrounding forest of North Lake. South Lake features a parking lot, a beach, and a rentable picnic pavilion, but is open for day use only. North Lake also includes a day-use area, with a beach, picnic tables, fireplaces, charcoal grills, and its own pavilion. Both beaches are pleasant and well maintained

RATINGS

Beauty: ✿ ✿ ✿ ✿
Privacy: ✿ ✿ ✿
Quiet: ✿ ✿ ✿
Cleanliness: ✿ ✿ ✿ ✿
Security: ✿ ✿ ✿ ✿
Spaciousness: ✿ ✿ ✿ ✿

and allow swimming from Memorial Day to Labor Day, but only when lifeguards are on duty.

The campground is separated into seven one-way loops, four of which border the shores of the lake. Be aware that not all loops may be open early and late in the season, and each loop will offer a slightly different experience depending on its size and location. Loops 2, 4, and 7 do not have lakefront sites but tend to be quieter, with Loop 7 being the most private. The largest is Loop 3, which offers a limited number of handicap-accessible sites. Loop 5 includes some of the best sites in the campground, particularly 145 through 148, which are footsteps from the water's edge.

Each loop is equipped with at least one comfort station with flush toilets and multiple water sources. Hot showers are a short walk away at the North Lake day-use area. The well-maintained and exceptionally clean facilities are worth the occasional inconvenience caused by construction and maintenance projects. At the exit of the campground are a trailer dump station and a trash and recycling center, making disposal of waste an easy task.

Unsurprisingly, lakefront sites tend to be the most popular, but all sites are heavily wooded, offering adequate privacy. Reservations are recommended at all times and necessary during summer weekends and holidays, with a two-night minimum stay required. Book early to obtain a lakefront site: it is well worth the effort. Sites are designated for tents and trailers only, with a pull-through parking area (two vehicles and two tents maximum), picnic table, and fire ring. There are no full-service sites in the campground, so RVs are few and far between. Rangers regularly patrol the grounds and quiet hours are strictly enforced from 10 p.m. to 7 a.m.

The popularity of the campground allows for a wide variety of organized activities. From late June to Labor Day, the posted *Wilderness Times* includes times and information on all group activities, from nature hikes to crafts, games, and live entertainment.

Fishing is permitted, and anglers can find a number of species in the lake, including brown bullhead, largemouth bass, chain pickerel, and pumpkinseed. No

KEY INFORMATION

ADDRESS:	P.O. Box 347, County Route 18 Haines Falls, NY 12436
OPERATED BY:	New York State Department of Environmental Conservation
INFORMATION:	(518) 589-5058; www.dec.state.ny .us/website/do/ca mping
OPEN:	Early May–late October
SITES:	219
EACH SITE HAS:	Picnic table and fire ring
ASSIGNMENT:	Choose from available sites or reservations
REGISTRATION:	On arrival or by reservation (reserve minimum 2 nights)
FACILITIES:	Water, flush toilets, showers
PARKING:	At site, maximum 2 vehicles
FEE:	$18/night
ELEVATION:	2,250 feet
RESTRICTIONS:	*Pets:* Dogs on leash with proof of currently valid rabies vaccination *Fires:* In fire rings only *Alcohol:* Prohibited *Vehicles:* Pop-up campers allowed *Other:* Quiet hours 10 p.m.–7 a.m. *Reservations:* 2-night stay required

MAP

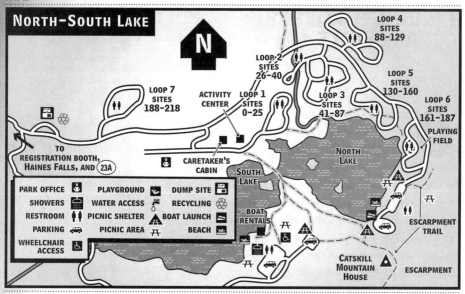

NORTH–SOUTH LAKE

LOOP 4 SITES 88–129

LOOP 2 SITES 26–40

LOOP 5 SITES 130–160

LOOP 7 SITES 188–218

ACTIVITY CENTER

LOOP 1 SITES 0–25

LOOP 3 SITES 41–87

LOOP 6 SITES 161–187

PLAYING FIELD

TO REGISTRATION BOOTH, HAINES FALLS, AND 23A

CARETAKER'S CABIN

SOUTH LAKE

NORTH LAKE

ESCARPMENT TRAIL

PARK OFFICE		PLAYGROUND		DUMP SITE
SHOWERS		WATER ACCESS		RECYCLING
RESTROOM		PICNIC SHELTER		BOAT LAUNCH
PARKING		PICNIC AREA		BEACH
WHEELCHAIR ACCESS				

BOAT RENTALS

CATSKILL MOUNTAIN HOUSE

ESCARPMENT

GETTING THERE

From I-87 (New York State Thruway), take NY 32 North for 6 miles to NY 32A. Follow NY 32A briefly to NY 23A West. In Haines Falls, turn right on CR 18. Drive 2 miles to the campground.

GPS COORDINATES

PARK ENTRANCE:

UTM Zone (WGS84)   18T
Easting   576882
Northing   4672142
Latitude   N 42°11'52"
Longitude   W 74°04'08"

motorboats are allowed, but rental rowboats, canoes, kayaks, and paddleboats are available. A paved boat ramp can be accessed at the North Lake day-use area.

More than any other campground in the region, North-South Lake offers the outdoor enthusiast a variety of hiking trails, including the well-traveled Escarpment Trail, Rock Shelter Trail, Mary's Glen Trail, and Schutt Road Trail. Artists' Rock lies about a half mile from the campground along the Escarpment Trail and is just one of many spots for picturesque views. Farther along Escarpment is North Point, where even the hardiest day hikers usually turn around. Alligator Rock (featuring "teeth" added by visitors over the years) is a favorite spot for families with small children. The now-vacant sites of the once-lavish 19th-century Kaaterskill Hotel and Catskill Mountain House are also easy to reach, and serve as a reminder of the area's rich history as a 200-year-old vacation destination.

For a community camping experience, North-South Lake is a fantastic campground during the summer. But for a quieter visit, consider a visit in the spring or fall (when the Catskills' autumn foliage at its peak).

11
TACONIC STATE PARK:
COPAKE FALLS AREA

ON THE EASTERN EDGE of the Hudson Valley, hugging the borders of Massachusetts and Connecticut, Taconic State Park stretches for nearly 15 miles along a thin line through the Taconic Mountains, broken only occasionally by privately held land. There are two separate campgrounds in Taconic State Park. On its southern end is the Rudd Pond Area, which consists of a narrow lake and an even narrower clearing with compact camping sites. The open field of that campground seems more an afterthought, and in stark contrast to the nicely shaded campground found at the Copake Falls Area on the park's northern end. For exploring the region, Copake Falls is the ideal place to pitch a tent.

As you enter the Copake Falls Area, it's easy to feel as if you've come upon a family summer camp. Groups of bikers crisscross the road in front of the Depot Deli, a popular lunch destination and store, which is directly across from the campground entrance. Just through the park gates on the left side of the road is a shallow pond that swarms with small children on hot summer days. Connected to this wading pool is what appears to be a small lake. It is actually a former mining pit filled with water. Known (appropriately enough) as Ore Pit Pond, it is spring-fed and reaches depths of 40 feet. Although there is no beach, a sturdy dock skirts the edge of the water. Both the wading pool and Ore Pit Pond open for weekend swimming on Memorial Day, then expand to weekday use at the end of June, and finally close on Labor Day. From 11 a.m. to 7 p.m., swimming is allowed, and both locals and campers take advantage.

Farther along the road are the park's remaining day-use facilities, including picnic tables, grills, comfort stations, showers, and a baseball diamond—all situated for easy access from a large parking lot. A nature center,

> *It's easy to feel as if you've come upon a family summer camp.*

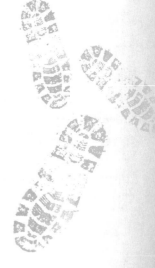

RATINGS

Beauty: ✿ ✿ ✿
Privacy: ✿ ✿
Quiet: ✿ ✿ ✿
Cleanliness: ✿ ✿ ✿
Security: ✿ ✿ ✿
Spaciousness: ✿ ✿ ✿

ADDRESS: Route 344
P.O. Box 100
Copake Falls, NY
12517

OPERATED BY: New York State
Office of Parks,
Recreation and His-
toric Preservation

INFORMATION: 518-329-3993;
nysparks.state.ny.us

OPEN: Early May–early
December

SITES: 46 tent, 24 tent-
platform, and
36 trailer sites

EACH SITE HAS: Picnic table and fire
ring with grate

ASSIGNMENT: Choose from
available sites or
reservations

REGISTRATION: On arrival

FACILITIES: Water, pit and flush
toilets, showers, pay
phone, laundry

PARKING: At site, maximum
2 vehicles

FEE: $13/night (plus
$3/night on
Friday, Saturday,
and holidays)

ELEVATION: 786 feet

RESTRICTIONS: *Pets:* Dogs in D Area
only, on leash and
with proof of cur-
rently valid rabies
vaccination
Fires: In fire rings
only
Alcohol: At site
Vehicles: Up to 30 feet
Other: Quiet hours
10 p.m.–7 a.m.
Reservations: 2-night
stay required

just north of the parking lot, provides programs on Saturdays and Sundays for all ages. Little more than a cabin, the center is filled with animal skulls, interesting geologic samples, leaves from the park's variety of trees, topographic maps, and a large tree-trunk cutaway, the rings of which present a timeline of the park's history. Young naturalists will not be disappointed.

The campground itself is located at the end of the road to the east of the parking lot, nestled on a wooded slope. Towering hemlocks shade a collection of somewhat crowded sites in the center of the A Area. The campground was once even more congested, and in recent years the park has removed more than 15 sites. That may not seem obvious at first, but sites become more secluded in the B Area, located directly east and uphill along the campground road. B-64 is one of the better sites, a private and spacious spot that is often the first choice for tent campers. Platform sites are scattered throughout the A and B areas, and are often necessary, as some parts of the campground are steeper than others.

Dogs are allowed, but only in the D Area, which consists exclusively of combination trailer–tent sites. There are no electric or water hook-ups in the campground, but RVs are directed to the C Area at the northwest corner of the campground. The park supervisor told us that they may convert some of the tent sites to trailer sites in the future, but there will still be plenty of sites exclusively for tent camping.

In addition to the land encompassed by Taconic State Park, many trails stretch into the Berkshire Mountains in Massachusetts, and visitors to Copake Falls can easily walk over the border and visit Bash Bish Falls and Mount Washington State Forest. Bash Bish Falls is one of the most popular day hikes accessible from the campground, but campers can choose from more than 25 miles of hiking trails, ranging from easy to difficult.

Bike rentals are available just outside the campground entrance, where County Route 344 is bisected by the Harlem Valley Rail Trail, a flat, paved path for walkers, runners, and bikers. There are plans to

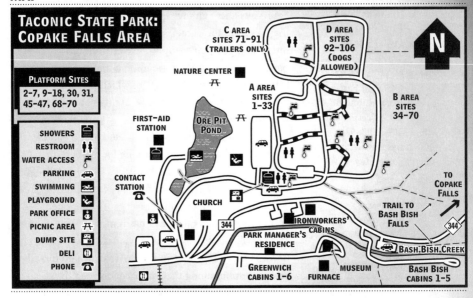

TACONIC STATE PARK:
COPAKE FALLS AREA

C AREA
SITES 71-91
(TRAILERS ONLY)

D AREA
SITES
92-106
(DOGS
ALLOWED)

N

NATURE CENTER

PLATFORM SITES
2-7, 9-18, 30, 31,
45-47, 68-70

A AREA
SITES
1-33

B AREA
SITES
34-70

FIRST-AID
STATION

ORE PIT
POND

SHOWERS
RESTROOM
WATER ACCESS
PARKING
SWIMMING
PLAYGROUND
PARK OFFICE
PICNIC AREA
DUMP SITE
DELI
PHONE

CONTACT
STATION

TO
COPAKE
FALLS

CHURCH

TRAIL TO
BASH BISH
FALLS

344

IRONWORKERS'
CABINS

PARK MANAGER'S
RESIDENCE

344

BASH BISH CREEK

GREENWICH
CABINS 1-6

MUSEUM

FURNACE

BASH BISH
CABINS 1-5

develop the Harley Valley Rail Trail so that it will one day stretch for 46 unbroken miles. Currently, some sections of the trail are not complete, but visitors can travel from one piece of the trail to the next along local roads through the rolling farmland. It is such a pleasure to drive on these roads, and exploring them at a slower pace on foot or bike makes for a lovely detour.

For people who do not find a few flaps of nylon to be adequate accommodations (surely not readers of this book), Copake Falls also has cabins. Iron ore was mined here for years, and the cabins are remnants of that time. Restored and available to rent, they are a unique alternative to a motel. You can learn more about the industrial history of the park at the Copake Iron Works Museum, a short distance down the road from the cabins.

The annual Falcon Ridge Folk Festival brings many campers to the park for the dancing and performances in nearby Hillsdale. Beyond Hillsdale, the surrounding area of Columbia County has a number of family activities, but the area's parks definitely offer enough to keep visitors busy for a weekend getaway or an entire week's vacation.

GETTING THERE

From Taconic State Parkway, take the Claverack/Hillsdale exit. Follow NY 23 East for 8 miles. In the village of Hillsdale, turn right on NY 22 South. Follow NY 22 South 4 miles. In the village of Copake Falls, turn left on CR 344 East. Follow CR 344 East for 0.5 miles; park entrance is on the left.

GPS COORDINATES

PARK ENTRANCE:
UTM Zone (WGS84)   18T
Easting   622405
Northing   4664220
Latitude   N 40°41'32"
Longitude   W 72°59'25"

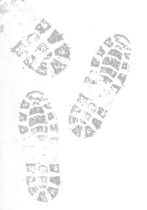

> *If you want to walk directly from your tent onto some of the most popular trails in the region, this is the campground for you.*

WHEN ONE SPEAKS OF HIKING in the Catskills, it is hard not to mention Slide Mountain. At 4,190 feet, it is the highest peak in the Catskills and the crown jewel of the Slide Mountain Wilderness, which makes up 47,500 acres of the park. Woodland Valley Campground is in the heart of this forest, and since great hiking abounds in this neck of the woods, it services backpackers and families alike. Sure, the more spacious Kenneth Wilson campground is only 13 miles away, and is a nice place to start your explorations of the central Catskills. But if you want to walk directly from your tent onto some of the most popular trails in the region (and back after a long day or two in the woods), Woodland Valley is the campground for you.

As you approach the campground, the northern side of the road is where you'll find the park ranger's office, a comfort station, the day-use parking area, and trailheads for both the Slide-Wittenberg Trail and the Woodland Valley–Denning Trail (which leads to the Giant Ledge–Slide Mountain Trail). These hikes, leading up both sides of the steep valley, are quite popular. The day-use area can fill up, with parking areas sometimes overflowing on very busy weekends. If you want to tackle Slide Mountain or other peaks, such as Wittenberg, Panther, Terrace, or Cornell, it's worth the few extra dollars to reserve a campsite at Woodland Valley, guaranteeing you a parking spot and an early-morning start.

Featuring two strips of standard sites divided by Woodland Valley Road, the campground can seem a little cramped and close to traffic. But the road comes to a dead end just past the western edge of the campground, so you need not worry about any cars passing through and disturbing the quiet. The campground also lacks power hookups, and many of the sites do not

RATINGS

Beauty: ☆ ☆ ☆ ☆
Privacy: ☆ ☆ ☆
Quiet: ☆ ☆ ☆
Cleanliness: ☆ ☆ ☆
Security: ☆ ☆ ☆
Spaciousness: ☆ ☆ ☆

have parking areas large enough to fit even a trailer, so tents are definitely in the majority.

Make sure to sign in at the campground office, located near the center of the campground adjacent to a shower house, recycling center, and dump station. Most of the sites are on the southern edge of Woodland Valley Road, bordering Woodland Valley Stream. Sites 1 through 15 are rather congested, so when making a reservation (recommended on weekends and holidays), choose sites in the 20s and 30s for their privacy. Site 25, sitting next to the rocky stream on a spur from the camp road, is perhaps the most desired. On the opposite side of Woodland Valley Road are sites 50 through 69, which skirt the edge of cliffs and are farther from the crowd, but also farther from the pleasant sound of the water.

Woodland Valley Stream, a tributary of Esopus Creek, occasionally dries up, but when running, it offers fishing for three types of trout. The camp staff discourages swimming and wading, as no area in the campground is designated for such use, so use your best judgment if you decide to enter the water. Nearby Kenneth Wilson Campground has a lake offering a sandy beach and boat rentals. Use your camping receipt to gain free access to its facilities during the length of your stay at Woodland Valley.

Some campers bike the 6 miles into Phoenecia along the windy Woodland Valley Road. In this small resort town, you'll easily find camp supplies, antiques stores, restaurants, and gift shops. An interesting sight is the line that can form in the evening at the town's one pay phone: cell phone reception is especially poor in the valley. At the edge of town is a large RV park that draws the more motorized crowd.

Whether you're staying in a tent, an RV, or a bed-and-breakfast, there are a number of popular tourist activities in the area. Tubing in Esopus Creek is the perfect way to stay cool during hot summer days. Local outfitters will supply transportation, flotation, and safety gear. The Catskill Mountain Railroad offers scenic rides and a rail shuttle to transport tubers upstream. The historic rail route also provides a fall-foliage route for the many leaf-peepers who drop by for the autumn colors.

KEY INFORMATION

ADDRESS:	1319 Woodland Valley Road Phoenecia, NY 12464
OPERATED BY:	New York State Department of Environmental Conservation
INFORMATION:	845-688-7647; www.dec.state.ny.us/website/do/camping
OPEN:	Mid-May–mid-October
SITES:	72
EACH SITE HAS:	Picnic table and fire ring
ASSIGNMENT:	Choose from available sites or reservations
REGISTRATION:	On arrival
FACILITIES:	Water, flush toilets, hot showers, pay phone
PARKING:	At site, maximum 2 vehicles
FEE:	$16/night
ELEVATION:	1,368 feet
RESTRICTIONS:	*Pets:* Dogs on leash with proof of currently valid rabies vaccination *Fires:* In fire rings only *Alcohol:* At site *Vehicles:* Up to 30 feet *Other:* Quiet hours 10 p.m.–7 a.m. *Reservations:* 2-night stay required

MAP

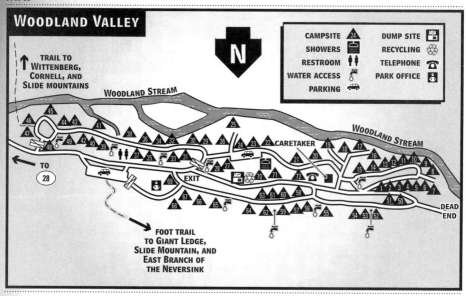

WOODLAND VALLEY

TRAIL TO WITTENBERG, CORNELL, AND SLIDE MOUNTAINS

WOODLAND STREAM

WOODLAND STREAM

CAMPSITE ▲24	DUMP SITE
SHOWERS	RECYCLING
RESTROOM	TELEPHONE ☎
WATER ACCESS	PARK OFFICE
PARKING 🚗	

CARETAKER

TO 28

EXIT

DEAD END

FOOT TRAIL TO GIANT LEDGE, SLIDE MOUNTAIN, AND EAST BRANCH OF THE NEVERSINK

GETTING THERE

From I-87 (New York State Thruway), take Exit 19, Kingston, to NY 28 West. Follow NY 28 West for 26 miles. In Phoenecia, just before a bridge and railroad tracks, turn left on Woodland Valley Road/High Street. Follow Woodland Valley Road/ High Street for 6 miles; campground entrance is on the left.

GPS COORDINATES

PARK ENTRANCE:
UTM Zone (WGS84)   18T
Easting   552785
Northing   4653929
Latitude   N 42°02'08"
Longitude   W 74°21'44"

Still, hiking is what this area is known for. Even when going for only a short walk in the woods, be sure to consult the park ranger for information on local trails and conditions. Use common sense to avoid getting lost in the woods, and always carry some basic supplies, such as water, snacks, extra clothing, and first-aid supplies. Remember that conditions on mountaintops and at night can vary drastically from those on the valley floor and during the day. A topographic map is a great help for visualizing the different elevations you may encounter on the trail.

Even if you don't take advantage of the many trails in the area, do take a moment to look at an area map. A meteor impact 350 million years ago left an outline of an almost-perfect circle around what is now Panther Mountain. This ring is nearly 7 miles across and clearly marked by Esopus Creek and Woodland Valley Stream. What was once a sunken meteor site is now one of the highest mountains in the Catskills, overlooking nicely wooded land with some of the best hiking in New York.

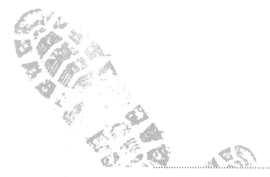

CENTRAL/LEATHERSTOCKING
AND CAPITAL

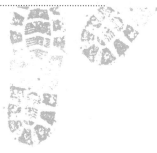

13
BOWMAN LAKE
STATE PARK

BOWMAN LAKE STATE PARK advertises itself as a "camper's paradise"—an exaggerated claim perhaps, but not entirely inaccurate. Open year-round for camping, it has 198 campsites, including 40 designated for tents only. Quaint signposts throughout the park have been constructed from rough-hewn wood and bespeak a commitment to providing a natural experience. Trees are thick, from maples and beech to cherry, pine, and dogwood. And ferns abound on the forest floor. It may not be located in the nearly boundless wilderness of the Adirondacks or Catskills, but it often seems like it.

Located about 30 miles north of Binghamton, Bowman Lake State Park was opened in the 1960s. Since then, it has strived to provide campers from central New York with a more private alternative to Gilbert Lake, Oquagua Creek, Chenango Valley, and other state parks in the region. But it is not some tiny hideaway, where there is nothing to do but pitch a tent. At 653 acres, it is a smaller park, but its facilities are the size of many larger parks. It has the proverbial beach and miles of trails to explore. Snicker if you like at the signs with raccoons on them that say, "I'm cute and I bite. And I may have rabies." But it's a good reminder that this is the wild—you will be sharing the park with animals, and you should respect any advice the experienced staff provides.

The campground is arranged in a series of overlapping loops, which can make for a confusing drive when trying to find your site. Yet it gives each site a unique vantage point. Sites 156 through 161 and 167 through 199 (including the wheelchair-accessible sites 193 through 195) have been established as tent-only. Sites 162 through 166 are no longer used and therefore have disappeared from the campground map. After all, with almost 200 sites to choose from, why worry about

> *Keep an eye out for white-tailed deer, red foxes, woodchucks, beavers, and a wide variety of birds.*

RATINGS

Beauty: ☆ ☆ ☆
Privacy: ☆ ☆ ☆ ☆
Quiet: ☆ ☆ ☆ ☆
Cleanliness: ☆ ☆ ☆ ☆
Security: ☆ ☆ ☆
Spaciousness: ☆ ☆ ☆ ☆

ADDRESS: 745 Bliven Sherman Road
Oxford, NY 13830

OPERATED BY: New York State Office of Parks, Recreation and Historic Preservation

INFORMATION: (607) 334-2718; nysparks.state.ny.us

OPEN: All year

SITES: 189

EACH SITE HAS: Picnic table and fire ring

ASSIGNMENT: Choose from available sites or reservations

REGISTRATION: On arrival or by reservation (reserve minimum 2 nights)

FACILITIES: Water, flush toilets, showers, pay phone

PARKING: At site, maximum 2 vehicles, or designated lot for hike-in and boat-in sites

FEE: $13/night (plus $3/night for Friday, Saturday, and holidays)

ELEVATION: 1,685 feet

RESTRICTIONS: *Pets:* Dogs on leash with proof of currently valid rabies vaccination
Fires: In fire rings only
Alcohol: At site
Vehicles: Up to 40 feet
Other: Quiet hours 10 p.m.–7 a.m.
Reservations: 2-night stay required

missing a few? Worriers can instead take this advice: There is little reason to reserve sites 156 through 161. They seem as if they've been tacked on, distributed along the edges of parking lots—not technically designated as overflow but not technically appealing, either.

Sites 167 through 199 occupy a small private loop on the southern edge of the campground, directly past the park office and near the shower building and a small playground. As much as we applaud the park for providing these tent-only sites, you may want to choose a site elsewhere, especially during the week or in the off-season when RVs are not choking the campground roads: the general sites tend to be larger and are often set back deep into the trees. Sites located at forks in the road (such as 55) will see a bit too much traffic, but those along the outer edges (including 17 and 18) are wonderfully private. Sites 124 through 155, on the campground's northern edge, are more open and less appealing. Comfort stations, dumpsters, and water spigots are scattered logically, so you need not worry about their proximity when choosing a site.

There is plenty to keep campers occupied in the park. A beach, basketball court, nature center, and a handful of swing sets will attract the kids. Motorboats are not permitted on 35-acre Bowman Lake, but kayaks, canoes, and rowboats are available to rent from the boathouse. If you plan to bring your own, make sure to obtain a permit from the park office. For a short walk, follow the small nature-trail loop around the lake and keep an eye out for white-tailed deer, red foxes, woodchucks, beavers, and a wide variety of birds. The park is a favorite of the Chenango Bird Club, which maintains an inventory of the avian population.

For more extended hikes, set off on the two cross-country ski trails in the park (2 and 3 miles long), or the Kopac Trail, a 5-mile loop that passes by nearby Whaley Pond and Kopac Pond. The Finger Lakes Trail, a 560-mile thoroughfare that runs along the southern edge of the state from the Alleghenies to the Catskills, makes an appearance in the park, winding its way along the shore of Bowman Lake itself. Outside the park's boundaries, the state Department of Environmental Conservation maintains 11,000 acres

MAP

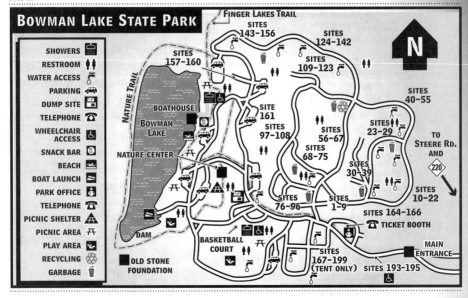

BOWMAN LAKE STATE PARK

Legend:
- SHOWERS
- RESTROOM
- WATER ACCESS
- PARKING
- DUMP SITE
- TELEPHONE
- WHEELCHAIR ACCESS
- SNACK BAR
- BEACH
- BOAT LAUNCH
- PARK OFFICE
- TELEPHONE
- PICNIC SHELTER
- PICNIC AREA
- PLAY AREA
- RECYCLING
- GARBAGE

FINGER LAKES TRAIL
SITES 143–156
SITES 124–142
SITES 109–123
SITES 157–160
NATURE TRAIL
BOATHOUSE
BOWMAN LAKE
NATURE CENTER
SITE 161
SITES 97–108
SITES 56–67
SITES 68–75
SITES 40–55
SITES 23–29
SITES 30–39
SITES 76–96
SITES 1–9
SITES 10–22
SITES 164–166
TICKET BOOTH
TO STEERE RD. AND 220
DAM
OLD STONE FOUNDATION
BASKETBALL COURT
SITES 167–199 (TENT ONLY)
SITES 193–195
MAIN ENTRANCE

N

---

of forested land, where even more adventures await outdoor enthusiasts.

Both the park and the campground are open year-round. Hunting is permitted in certain corners, so hikers should make sure to wear brightly colored clothing during hunting seasons and should always stay on the trails. In the wintertime, local cross-country skiers and snowmobilers descend on the park. Central New York is legendary for its heavy snowfall. Keep that in mind if you are one of those hardier souls who enjoy winter camping. Only a handful of sites (1 through 4 and 76 through 82) are available from November through March, but it will hardly be a problem to book one.

In the nearby village of Oxford, which was known for its bluestone mining in the 1800s, you can grab lunch, shop for antiques, and even catch a folk-music performance at the Night Eagle Cafe. However, it is likely that you will not even need to leave the park, especially in the summer when the concession stand is selling camping supplies. Whether you will find it "paradise" or not, though, is up to you.

GETTING THERE

From NY 17 West, take NY 12 North and follow it to Oxford. Turn left on CR 220 West. Follow CR 220 for about 6 miles to Steere Road. Stay straight on Steere Road for 1 mile and follow signs to park entrance.

GPS COORDINATES

PARK ENTRANCE:

UTM Zone (WGS84)	18T
Easting	444248
Northing	4707330
Latitude	N 42°30'59"
Longitude	W 75°40'43"

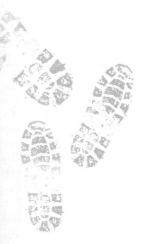

A splendid place to pitch a tent—serene, private, and little known in camping circles.

RATINGS

Beauty: ✪ ✪ ✪ ✪ ✪
Privacy: ✪ ✪ ✪
Quiet: ✪ ✪ ✪ ✪ ✪
Cleanliness: ✪ ✪ ✪ ✪
Security: ✪ ✪ ✪
Spaciousness: ✪ ✪ ✪

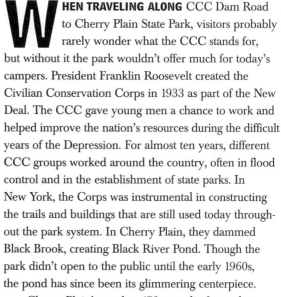

WHEN TRAVELING ALONG CCC Dam Road to Cherry Plain State Park, visitors probably rarely wonder what the CCC stands for, but without it the park wouldn't offer much for today's campers. President Franklin Roosevelt created the Civilian Conservation Corps in 1933 as part of the New Deal. The CCC gave young men a chance to work and helped improve the nation's resources during the difficult years of the Depression. For almost ten years, different CCC groups worked around the country, often in flood control and in the establishment of state parks. In New York, the Corps was instrumental in constructing the trails and buildings that are still used today throughout the park system. In Cherry Plain, they dammed Black Brook, creating Black River Pond. Though the park didn't open to the public until the early 1960s, the pond has since been its glimmering centerpiece.

Cherry Plain's modest 176 acres lie fewer than 20 miles east of Albany. Yet the park seems much farther from the capital, hidden away down country roads just north of the Taconic Valley, along the border with Massachusetts and Vermont. Only 20 sites make up the entire campground, and almost all have views of the quiet Black River Pond. For such a small park with a carry-in-carry-out policy, you may not expect too many amenities. But this is no primitive campground—comfort stations with running water and water spigots are found in each of the two camping sections. A shower facility is available, and firewood is for sale at the registration booth for $5/bundle.

The first group of sites is so pleasant that when we visited our first impression was that they must be the tent sites. Surprisingly, they are reserved primarily for trailers, but we figure RVs and pop-ups sometimes deserve nice scenery too. Pine trees cast ample shade upon these nine sites, but they are a bit close together.

A small stream runs along the edge of the section, with a charming wooden bridge crossing over it near site 1. Between sites 2 and 3 is the car-top boat launch, with a tiny dock. Sites 1 through 4 skirt the water's edge, and sites 5 through 9 are not far from the pond.

Tent campers will likely opt for the other section, which is truly separate from the RVs and consists only of walk-in sites. No vehicles are allowed here, but this does not necessarily mean that people will not haul all sorts of camping equipment (from hibachis to lawn chairs and inflatable boats) the short distance from their parked cars. After passing through the day-use area, the first sites in the group (11 through 13) open up to the camp road and sit upon a small ledge. There are some views of the water, but unless horseshoes is your game (there is a horseshoe pit nearby), take a pass on these and drive to the parking lot just past site 13.

From the lot, a short path goes downhill past five well-wooded sites to the water, then back uphill to a comfort station and two more sites; you can return to the lot along a service road. The closest site is 14, about a 15-yard walk on the well-maintained path. Sites 15 and 20 are the two nearest the comfort station, convenient to be sure, but also a bit too far from the water's edge. Sites 16 through 19 are all directly on the water, with 18 and 19 offering the most privacy. While there are not many sites to go around, this is a splendid place to pitch a tent—serene, private, and little-known in camping circles. It is among the nicest spots in all of New York state.

Between the two camping sections is a sandy beach with picnic pavilion. Swimmers enjoy the cool water of Black River Pond from late June to Labor Day, when lifeguards are on duty. Fishermen come for the bass, bullhead, and pickerel. Visitors can rent rowboats and paddleboats, but will have to leave any motorboats at home. Canoes and kayaks are a common sight, and the occasional small sailboat can be seen searching for a breeze. At the far western end of the water, bring a chair to sit and overlook the dam's spillway, where you can crack open a book and spend a quiet summer day. Another park treat is the 1-mile hike to the Charcoal Kiln Site. Follow the signs from

KEY INFORMATION

ADDRESS:	26 State Park Road P.O. Box 11 Cherry Plain, NY 12040
OPERATED BY:	New York State Office of Parks, Recreation and Historic Preservation
INFORMATION:	(518) 733-5400; nysparks.state .ny.us
OPEN:	Early May–early October
SITES:	10 trailer and 10 tent
EACH SITE HAS:	Picnic table and fire ring
ASSIGNMENT:	Choose from available sites or reservations
REGISTRATION:	On arrival or by reservation (reserve minimum 2 nights)
FACILITIES:	Water, flush toilets, hot showers, pay phone
PARKING:	At site, maximum 2 vehicles
FEE:	$10/night (plus $3/night for Friday, Saturday, and holidays)
ELEVATION:	1,427 feet
RESTRICTIONS:	*Pets:* Dogs on leash with proof of currently valid rabies vaccination *Fires:* In fire rings only *Alcohol:* At site *Vehicles:* Up to 15 feet *Other:* Quiet hours 10 p.m.–7 a.m.; fires out by 11 p.m. *Reservations:* 2-night stay required

MAP

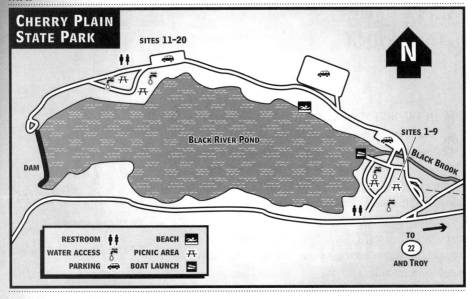

CHERRY PLAIN STATE PARK

SITES 11-20

N

BLACK RIVER POND

SITES 1-9

BLACK BROOK

DAM

RESTROOM 👫	BEACH 🏊
WATER ACCESS 🚰	PICNIC AREA 🏕
PARKING 🚐	BOAT LAUNCH 🛥

TO
22
AND TROY

GETTING THERE

From Interstate 87, take Exit 21A. Follow I-90 (Berkshire Spur) to Exit B3. Turn left on CR 22 North. Follow CR 22 for 20 miles. Turn left on CCC Dam Road. Follow CCC Dam Road 2.5 miles to park entrance on left.

GPS COORDINATES

PARK ENTRANCE:
UTM Zone (WGS84)   18T
Easting   630432
Northing   4720245
Latitude   N 42°37'25"
Longitude   W 73°24'34"

the main parking lot to see the remains of the stone oven where hardwoods were once covered with soil and set aflame. Deprived of oxygen, the resulting product, charcoal, was prized because it burns hotter and cleaner than wood.

Though the park is small in comparison to many others, there are plenty of recreational opportunities just beyond its borders. The Capital Region Wildlife Management Area surrounds Cherry Plain with more than 4,000 acres of land. If entering the park from the east, you may pass Black River Stables, which offer trail rides in the area, including some on bridle paths that pass through Cherry Plain.

Today many campers still appreciate the ease of charcoal. Especially on a rainy evening or after a long day, it can make for a fast and easy dinner. But few would disagree that one of the best things about camping is sitting around a campfire lit with real wood. Come to Cherry Plain in late September, when there's a nip in the air and autumn colors are bursting all around you, and you'll be happy you're here at the water's edge, beside a warm campfire, rather than home on the couch in front of the TV.

15
DELTA LAKE
STATE PARK

IN THE HISTORY-RICH Mohawk Valley, Delta Lake has quite a story of its own. It was once a natural lake, but when Ice Age glaciers covered the area and then retreated, it dried up. On the site of the ancient lakebed, the village of Delta was established and thrived, due in large part to its location on the Black River Canal, which was dug in the 1850s to connect the city of Rome to the Erie Canal. As the area grew, the need for a reservoir outweighed the need for a town. In 1912, the residents of Delta were relocated and the Mohawk River was dammed. A large body of water made a homecoming to the area after being gone for thousands of years, and now it had a name—Delta Lake. Fifty years passed before the state decided to create a park to take advantage of the recreational opportunities the reservoir offers. Go for a visit to Delta Lake State Park these days and, it is rumored, you may see rooftops of the flooded residences when the water level is low.

Lying on a peninsula that juts out from the southern shore, the park takes full advantage of its surrounding waters, including placing its campground directly on the lake. There is private development on other parts of the lake. Thankfully, it has not gotten out of hand, and although you can see some buildings along the shores, the views are still excellent. Entering the park, you pass the registration booth and then bear right to more than 100 camping sites.

Like most state-run campgrounds, Delta Lake State Park does not have electrical hookups, so some RV-ers may choose to motor on and plug in at the privately owned A-OK Campground and Marina on the north shore of the lake. Still, trailers and pop-ups are inevitable, especially since the campground is a pleasant, well-run facility. The park staff even has placed flower boxes on the classic hewn park signs. With so

> *Go for a visit to Delta Lake State Park these days and, it is rumored, you may see rooftops of the flooded residences when the water level is low.*

RATINGS

Beauty: ✿ ✿ ✿
Privacy: ✿ ✿
Quiet: ✿ ✿ ✿
Cleanliness: ✿ ✿ ✿
Security: ✿ ✿ ✿
Spaciousness: ✿ ✿ ✿

ADDRESS:	8797 State Route 46 Rome, NY 13440
OPERATED BY:	New York State Office of Parks, Recreation and Historic Preservation
INFORMATION:	(315) 337-4670; nysparks.state.ny.us
OPEN:	Early May–mid October
SITES:	101
EACH SITE HAS:	Picnic table and fire ring
ASSIGNMENT:	Choose from available sites or reservations
REGISTRATION:	On arrival or by reservation (reserve minimum 2 nights)
FACILITIES:	Water, flush toilets, hot showers, pay phone, laundry
PARKING:	At site, maximum 2 vehicles
FEE:	$13/night (plus $3/night for Friday, Saturday, and holidays)
ELEVATION:	555 feet
RESTRICTIONS:	*Pets:* Dogs on leash with proof of currently valid rabies vaccination *Fires:* In fire rings only *Alcohol:* At site *Vehicles:* Up to 40 feet *Other:* Quiet hours 10 p.m.–7 a.m. *Reservations:* 2-night stay required

many campgrounds in the state that look similar, sometimes it's the little things that make a difference.

Flat and made up of three main loops, the campground is located on a dead-end road. With a large proportion of waterfront sites available (nearly one out of every five), you have a good chance of landing a premium spot. No one waterfront site is better than any other, so choose from the following: 8, 10, 12, 14, 16, 18, 20, 45, 46, 48, 50, 51, 53, 86, 88, 90, 92, 94, or 95. These book up fast on weekends, but the water is still easily accessible from interior sites.

In all three loops, tall hardwoods form a shady canopy and act as adequate boundaries, but neighbors may be closer than some would wish. Loop A (sites 1 through 37) is the most exposed, with almost no understory to separate campers. Sites 38 through 70 make up Loop B. The center of this loop is a bit more cluttered, but more foliage sprouts from the forest floor, giving at least the feeling of privacy. Loop C (sites 71 through 101) is the smallest but also the most heavily wooded. Sure, Loop C has only one comfort station (the other loops have two), but being quietly tucked away at the end of the camp road, this loop is our favorite. Dumpsters are placed conveniently throughout all loops, and the shower building, on the camp road between Loops B and C, is a short walk from just about any site.

The popular day-use area is filled with picnic areas, parking lots, a swimming beach, and a lake overlook. You can be sure it will be busy on hot summer days. Trails in the park connect the campground to three tiny ponds and Treasure Island, a small chunk of land within spitting distance of the peninsula. A trailer boat launch is another big attraction, and anglers search the waters for bass, bullhead, northern pike, perch, trout, and walleye pike. The campground map helpfully includes locations where the various types of fish are commonly found and approximate depths of the water (65 feet at its deepest). All types of boats are allowed on the 2,560-acre lake, and if you have water access, you are welcome to launch canoes and kayaks directly from your site. Don't have a boat? Take a short drive to the previously mentioned A-OK Campground & Marina, where all varieties of watercraft are available for rent.

MAP

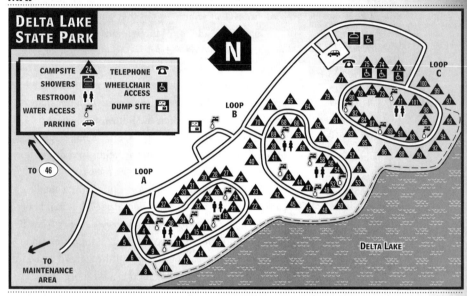

For a scenic view of the region, take a drive on the Black River Trail, a 111-mile byway that runs north along the western edge of the Adirondacks from Rome past Delta Lake to Ogdensburg on the St. Lawrence River. In the city of Rome, you can visit Fort Stanwix National Monument—the fort was built by the British during the French and Indian War and later occupied by Americans during the Revolutionary War. The fort protected the Oneida Carrying Place, a 3-mile portage between the Mohawk River and Wood Creek. It was an essential trail for transporting goods, news, and, unfortunately, diseases, as early travelers journeyed the Northeast's inland waterways. Today Fort Stanwix sits at a busy intersection, its simple log construction contrasting so sharply with the surrounding box stores and chain restaurants. It's a fascinating place to visit for an afternoon, and when you return to your tent at Delta Lake, you can rest assured that you will have you have a safe and pleasant place to spend the night.

GETTING THERE

Take I-90 (New York State Thruway) to Exit 32, Westmoreland/Rome. Follow NY 233 North to Rome. Then follow NY 46 North 6 miles to park entrance.

GPS COORDINATES

PARK ENTRANCE:

UTM Zone (WGS84)   18T

Easting   466330

Northing   4793133

Latitude   N 43°17'25"

Longitude   W 75°24'54"

16
FAIR HAVEN BEACH
STATE PARK

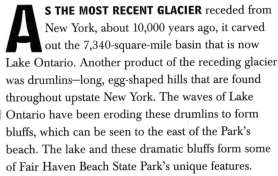

> *Enjoy scenic family camping along Lake Ontario.*

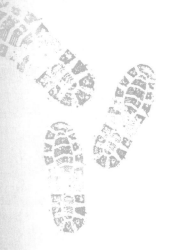

AS THE MOST RECENT GLACIER receded from New York, about 10,000 years ago, it carved out the 7,340-square-mile basin that is now Lake Ontario. Another product of the receding glacier was drumlins—long, egg-shaped hills that are found throughout upstate New York. The waves of Lake Ontario have been eroding these drumlins to form bluffs, which can be seen to the east of the Park's beach. The lake and these dramatic bluffs form some of Fair Haven Beach State Park's unique features.

Lake Ontario forms Fair Haven Beach State Park's northern edge, and Little Sodus Bay the park's eastern boundary. Overnight docks and a public boat launch are available in Little Sodus Bay and provide boating access to Lake Ontario. The remainder of the park is bordered along its southern and western edges by Sterling Pond and Sterling Marsh. Given the quantity and diversity of the park's waterscape, fishing, boating, and birding make up the majority of activities available at the park. Swimming is allowed only in designated areas when a lifeguard is on duty.

The park has three separate campgrounds as well as 35 cabins and cottages that can be rented. Cabins and cottages are booked solid most of the season and require reservations far in advance. The Bluff camping area contains 44 large pull-up sites with electric hookups for RVs. The Lakeview camping area has 14 sites and can accommodate various RVs and trailers, but has no electric sites. The Drumlin camping area has 126 sites that range from tent-only sites to 30-foot RV/trailer sites; none have electric hookups.

The Bluff camping sites are essentially for RVs—they are surrounded by trees and have no views of the lake, pond, or marsh. The Lakeview sites sit atop the bluff and offer expansive views of Lake Ontario. The sites are closely spaced and consequently provide little

RATINGS

Beauty: ✿ ✿ ✿
Privacy: ✿ ✿ ✿
Quiet: ✿ ✿ ✿
Cleanliness: ✿ ✿ ✿
Security: ✿ ✿ ✿
Spaciousness: ✿ ✿ ✿

privacy. Both the Bluff and Lakeview sites have access to comfort stations and potable water but no showers. Campers interested in views of the lake should consider the Lakeview area, but the majority of sites for tent campers are in the Drumlin camping area.

A canopy of conifers and mixed hardwoods shades the Drumlin camping area, which is served by three comfort stations with showers. Potable-water stations are available throughout the area, as are a centrally located dumpster and recycling station. Sites along the outside western edge of the campground are shielded from the park's main road by a thin row of trees, and view of the park's waterscape are absent. Interior sites near the western edge are denser then those along the edge and also lack views of the waterscape. Though the surrounding understory is thick, brief glimpses of the pond and marsh are available to interior sites along the eastern edge. These sites are also fairly dense, though, and well within view of the nearby sites. The exterior loop of the campground road provides access to the more desirable sites, most of which are tent-only (with a few for small trailers). The loop road descends toward the marsh. This change in elevation, combined with the addition of a dense understory, isolates these sites along the eastern edge from the rest of the campground. Increased spaciousness, thicker woods, and greater distances between sites complement this privacy. Views of Sterling Marsh are greatly improved here with some sites lying on the water's edge. The last few sites along this loop share views of Sterling Pond as well as the marsh.

The park has numerous picnic tables, comfort stations, and grills for public use. Near the East Beach, look for a recreation hall, snack bar, bathhouse, camp store, and boat and bicycle rentals. Playgrounds and a ball field scattered throughout make this park very family friendly. Two short hiking trails are also available for those wishing to forgo the park's main activities. Wildlife in the area is most notably beaver, muskrat, a variety of waterfowl, and migratory birds; very fortunate visitors might catch a glimpse of an otter.

Wildlife enthusiasts and hikers looking for more-remote trails should visit Sterling Lakeshore Park and

KEY INFORMATION

ADDRESS:	Route 104A, P.O. Box 16 Fair Haven, NY 13064
OPERATED BY:	New York State Office of Parks, Recreation and Historic Preservation
INFORMATION:	(315) 947-5205; nysparks.state.ny.us
OPEN:	Early April–mid-October
SITES:	185 tent sites, 46 electric sites
EACH SITE HAS:	Picnic table and fire ring
ASSIGNMENT:	Choose from available sites or reservations
REGISTRATION:	3 p.m.–9 p.m.
FACILITIES:	Picnic areas, pavilion, potable water, flush toilets, park store, boat launch, showers
PARKING:	At site
FEE:	$13/night most tent sites; add $3/night Friday, Saturday, and holidays
ELEVATION:	384 feet
RESTRICTIONS:	*Pets:* Dogs on leash with proof of currently valid rabies vaccination *Fires:* In fire rings only *Alcohol:* Allowed *Vehicles:* RVs and trailers limited to specific sites *Other:* Quiet hours 10 p.m.–7 a.m.; 6 people maximum/site; maximum 14-night stay *Reservations:* 2-night stay required

MAP

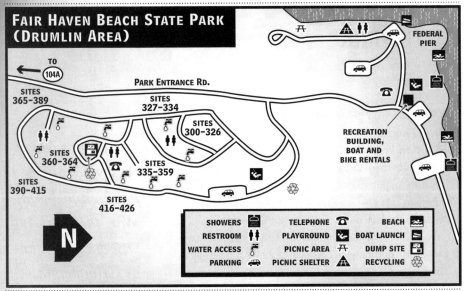

FAIR HAVEN BEACH STATE PARK (DRUMLIN AREA)

TO 104A

PARK ENTRANCE RD.

SITES 365–389

SITES 327–334

SITES 300–326

SITES 360–364

SITES 335–359

SITES 390–415

SITES 416–426

FEDERAL PIER

RECREATION BUILDING, BOAT AND BIKE RENTALS

N

SHOWERS	TELEPHONE ☎	BEACH
RESTROOM	PLAYGROUND	BOAT LAUNCH
WATER ACCESS	PICNIC AREA ⊼	DUMP SITE
PARKING	PICNIC SHELTER ⚠	RECYCLING ♻

GETTING THERE

From I-90 (New York State Thruway), take Exit 34A, I-481 North, toward Oswego. Follow I-481 for 6.7 miles until it changes to NY 481 North. Continue 20 miles and turn left on NY 176/NY 3. Follow NY 3 for 11.7 miles and turn left on NY 104A. Follow NY 104A for 4 miles. Park entrance is on the right.

GPS COORDINATES

PARK ENTRANCE:

UTM Zone (WGS84)   18T
Easting   362466
Northing   4797594
Latitude   N 43°19'07"
Longitude   W 76°41'46"

Nature Center, a short drive north from the park. This park also features glacial buffs and diverse waterscapes as well as guided nature walks.

Long-distance hikers and cyclists may want to try either the North Trail or the Hojak Trail, both of which are converted railroad beds and offer long and mostly flat routes. Access to both is within Fair Haven. Visitors during the summer may also want to consider the Sterling Renaissance Festival, open weekends from July to mid-August. Travelers wishing to view more of Lake Ontario—with its historic battlegrounds, forts, lighthouses, vineyards, and other attractions—can drive, bike, or walk along the Seaway Trail, a 454-mile byway that traverses the northern edge of New York state and offers a pleasant alternative to the interstate.

17
GLIMMERGLASS STATE PARK

THE FAMILY-FRIENDLY CAMPGROUND at Glimmerglass State Park lies in the heart of New York's Leatherstocking region, a hilly collection of farms and small towns named after James Fenimore Cooper's *Leatherstocking Tales,* which include *The Pioneers, The Deerslayer,* and, most famously, *The Last of the Mohicans.* In Cooper's classic stories, set during the French and Indian War, the sparkling Otsego Lake is known as Glimmerglass. Similar in shape and geology to the Finger Lakes, Otsego is long and narrow, cutting a sliver in the land for 8 miles. On the northern end of the lake is Glimmerglass State Park; at the southern end is Cooperstown, founded by and named after James Fenimore's father. Cooperstown, as most people know, is home to the Baseball Hall of Fame. Local lore tells how baseball was invented in the town, but the origins of the sport have been debated for years. Whatever the true story, the region offers a nice combination of history and recreation, and Glimmerglass is a fine place for tent campers to begin their explorations.

The manicured lawns and rolling hills of the park are home to two separate camping areas. Two loops make up the main camping area, with 37 standard, if a bit small, sites. Towering fir trees divide and shade the spaces, but there is no understory for privacy. A field separates the two loops, and on busy weekends children collect there to play and reach for the skies on the swing set. Crowds abate during the week, and walk-ins can easily find openings. Trailers are popular, but sites 25A and 23A are tent-only due to their small size. We prefer sites 20, 21, or the private 36 over the bare and exposed 33 through 35. The new comfort stations with showers are clean, well maintained, and located near the garbage and recycling centers. Follow campground procedures for refuse—raccoons are common in the park and not too picky about what they have for dinner.

> *In Cooper's classic stories, set during the French and Indian War, the sparkling Otsego Lake is known as Glimmerglass.*

RATINGS

Beauty: ☆ ☆ ☆
Privacy: ☆ ☆
Quiet: ☆ ☆ ☆
Cleanliness: ☆ ☆ ☆ ☆
Security: ☆ ☆ ☆
Spaciousness: ☆ ☆

ADDRESS: 1527 County Highway 31 Cooperstown, NY 13326

OPERATED BY: New York State Office of Parks, Recreation and Historic Preservation

INFORMATION: (607) 547-8662; nysparks.state.ny.us

OPEN: Mid-May–early October

SITES: 60 (20 nonreservable walk-in sites at Beaver Pond Area)

EACH SITE HAS: Picnic table, grill, and fire ring

ASSIGNMENT: Choose from available sites or reservations

REGISTRATION: On arrival or by reservation (reserve minimum 2 nights)

FACILITIES: Water, flush toilets, showers, pay phone (only pit toilet at walk-in sites)

PARKING: At site, maximum 2 vehicles, or central lot for walk-in sites

FEE: $13/night (plus $3/night for Friday, Saturday, and holidays)

ELEVATION: 1,276 feet

RESTRICTIONS: *Pets:* Dogs on leash with proof of currently valid rabies vaccination
Fires: In fire rings only
Alcohol: At site
Vehicles: Up to 30 feet
Other: Quiet hours 10 p.m.–8 a.m.
Reservations: 2-night stay required

Near Beaver Pond, on the northern end of the park, is the separate primitive-camping area. Reservations are not available for these 23 sites, but they fill up on weekends on a first-come, first-serve basis. Although there is no water and only pit toilets to use in this section, this is where you will find the majority of the tents in the park. Two of the most popular sites are 38 and 39, located directly on the edge of a small pond. Site 39 contains a lean-to, which doubles as a warming hut during the ice-skating season. Sites 40 through 49 feature low foliage, bushes, and small, young trees. While 40 through 43 are the most private and are restricted to tents and a single car per site, sites 46 and 48 offer the best shade.

Across from Beaver Pond, an open field hosts sites 50 through 60. Pop-ups are allowed in the field, and since these sites offer absolutely no privacy or shade, they are the least appealing of the bunch, even though it would not be a bad place to watch the sunset. Winter camping is allowed at Beaver Pond but is rare, according to camp staff (only three or four campers each season). Perhaps this would be a great place to try out cold-weather gear, but be sure to call ahead. If you decide to visit in the winter, the park's many activities include ice-skating, ice fishing, snowshoeing, cross-country skiing, and snow tubing.

In the warmer months, the beach is a big attraction. It has lifeguards, pavilion, picnic shelters, snack bar, first-aid station, ball fields, and playgrounds. There is a car-top boat launch at the park, and canoes and kayaks are a common sight, but those with larger vessels will have to go to Cooperstown for the trailer boat launch. Anglers can use the shoreline or boats to fish for lake and brown trout, smallmouth and largemouth bass, coho salmon, brown bullhead, yellow perch, or chain pickerel. Several trails loop through the park, including a short nature trail near Beaver Pond and the longer Woodland Trail, both of which attract birders and locals looking for an afternoon jaunt. The orange-blazed, 2.5-mile Sleeping Lion Trail, which starts behind Hyde Hall and leads to Mount Wellington, is named for what the peak is said to resemble from the south.

MAP

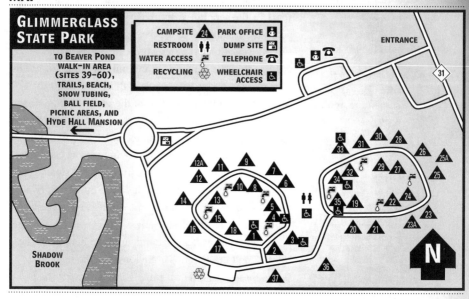

Within the park is a state historic site, consisting of Hyde Hall and its many outbuildings. The 50-room Classical Revival mansion is the centerpiece of a property once owned by George Clark. The state bought the land from his descendents in the 1960s. Today, visitors can tour Hyde Hall daily in the summer, but there is a $7 entrance fee.

If you are not game for a trip to the Baseball Hall of Fame, perhaps you would like to take in a little theater or opera before a night of camping. During July and August, the Leatherstocking Theatre Company is in residence at Hyde Hall for two productions. Just down the road on Route 80, the renowned Glimmerglass Opera holds shows at the Alice Busch Opera Theater four to five days a week during the summer. Make a full day of it and check other local attractions, such as the Fenimore Art Museum, Farmers' Museum, and Ommegang Brewery.

Glimmerglass has much to offer campers. Even if you're not an adventurer on par with Cooper's famed character Hawkeye, this bit of central New York is a fine getaway for a family looking for a bit of fresh air.

GETTING THERE

From I-90 (New York State Thruway), take Exit 25A to I-88. Follow I-88 to Exit 24, Duanesburg-Cooperstown. Follow NY 20 West for approximately 36 miles. In the town of East Springfield, take a left on CR 31 South. Follow CR 31 South 4 miles to park entrance on right.

GPS COORDINATES

PARK ENTRANCE:

UTM Zone (WGS84)	18T
Easting	511338
Northing	4736998
Latitude	N 42°47'08"
Longitude	W 74°51'41"

18

Fayetteville

> *The two lakes found in the park are actually green.*

THE FIRST THING THAT SURPRISES many visitors to Green Lakes State Park is the fact that its name is neither an exaggeration nor a quaint evocation of the surrounding wilderness, but an accurate description of the water: the two lakes found in the park are actually green. The smaller one is Round Lake, an almost perfect circle of emerald water surrounded by heavily wooded slopes. The larger one is Green Lake—about twice its neighbor's size and also round, but with a long spur that juts out and ends at a sandy beach. Formed by Ice Age glaciers about 14,000 years ago, both are meromictic, a rare type of lake (there are only a few others in the United States) where the surface and bottom waters do not mix. They are small, but astoundingly deep—it's nearly 200 feet to the bottom of each! These factors, along with the presence of calcium carbonate, cause mainly green light to be reflected by the water, producing the odd but beautiful color that intrigues and delights those who take to the trails along the lakes' shores.

The lakes are indeed gorgeous. We wish we could say the same about the park's campground. Divided into two looping sections, the sites at Green Lakes are grassy, clean, and adequately large, but they are also poorly shaded and offer little privacy. The first section along the camp road is known as Pine Wood, which is not the most accurate name. There are pine trees on the far edges of sites 1 through 64, but none dividing them. The second section, Rolling Hills, is more aptly named and contains sites 65 through 132. Exterior sites are set upon grassy slopes and often overlook the mix of tents and RVs that fill up the campground. Electric sites make up the northern end of each section. When placing a reservation, which you will need on summer weekends, skip those and opt for any site where fewer neighboring sites are reserved. This seems obvious, but we say it

RATINGS

Beauty: ✿ ✿
Privacy: ✿ ✿
Quiet: ✿ ✿ ✿
Cleanliness: ✿ ✿ ✿
Security: ✿ ✿ ✿ ✿
Spaciousness: ✿ ✿

because no particular site stands out, and you are most likely to enjoy your stay if you have more privacy.

The campground features the typical amenities, including large comfort stations, conveniently distributed water spigots, and even small jungle gyms in the center of each section. A nature center in the Pine Wood section is open throughout the summer and offers programs for youngsters. And just south of Pine Wood, a series of eight rustic cabins are available to rent. They are nothing fancy, but a few are set along the edge of a cliff and look down onto the waters of Round Lake.

We don't mean to paint the campground as inadequate, but compared with the rest of the park, it is the place where you will want to spend the least amount of time. Green Lakes is quite simply one of the nicest parks in the New York system—it certainly has the best outdoor facilities and presents the best range of activities in the Syracuse area.

The lakes are, of course, the stars of the park. The beach entices locals on summer days and is worth visiting, but you will first want to take a stroll along the trails that follow the lakes' outer rims. The water is very dangerous away from the beach. Take the NO SWIMMING signs seriously and keep your feet on the impeccably maintained path. This is where the local high school's cross-country team trains in the summer and where many a dog walker comes to escape the bland, paved roads of the suburbs—and for good reason. As the trail approaches the water's edge, notice how the shore drops off suddenly, almost as if it were a bottomless pit. Native Americans and early European settlers believed just that. Scientists still study the lower depths, where evidence of ancient plants and animals may exist.

There is more to the park, though, than just the lakes. Make sure to stop by the campground office and pick up a map to the park's 10 miles of trails. A trail leaving from Pine Wood and through Rolling Hills will take you south down a hill and into the surrounding woods, some of the only old-growth forest in the region. Follow another trail west from Rolling Hills and you will find yourself among the rolling fields of Farmer's Hill. This is the site of a former farm and was

KEY INFORMATION

ADDRESS:	7900 Green Lakes Road Fayetteville, NY 13066
OPERATED BY:	New York State Office of Parks, Recreation and Historic Preservation
INFORMATION:	(315) 637-6111; nysparks.state.ny.us
OPEN:	Late-May–early October
SITES:	132
EACH SITE HAS:	Picnic table and fire ring
ASSIGNMENT:	Choose from available sites or reservations
REGISTRATION:	On arrival or by reservation (reserve minimum 2 nights)
FACILITIES:	Water, flush toilets, hot showers, pay phone
PARKING:	At site, maximum 2 vehicles
FEE:	$13/night (plus $3/night for Fridays, Saturdays, and holidays)
ELEVATION:	469 feet
RESTRICTIONS:	*Pets:* Dogs on leash with proof of currently valid rabies vaccination *Fires:* In fire rings only *Alcohol:* At site *Vehicles:* Up to 40 feet *Other:* Quiet hours 10 p.m.–7 a.m.; no private boats on lakes; swimming allowed from Memorial Day to Labor Day *Reservations:* 2-night stay required

MAP

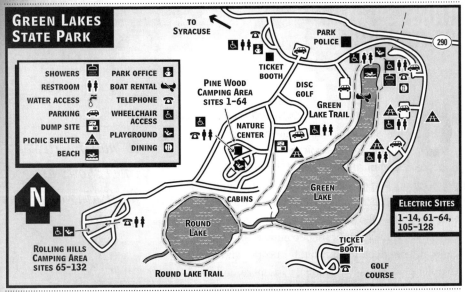

GREEN LAKES STATE PARK

Legend:
- SHOWERS
- RESTROOM
- WATER ACCESS
- PARKING
- DUMP SITE
- PICNIC SHELTER
- BEACH
- PARK OFFICE
- BOAT RENTAL
- TELEPHONE
- WHEELCHAIR ACCESS
- PLAYGROUND
- DINING

TO SYRACUSE

PARK POLICE

290

TICKET BOOTH

PINE WOOD CAMPING AREA SITES 1-64

DISC GOLF

GREEN LAKE TRAIL

NATURE CENTER

N

CABINS

GREEN LAKE

ROUND LAKE

ELECTRIC SITES
1-14, 61-64, 105-128

ROLLING HILLS CAMPING AREA SITES 65-132

TICKET BOOTH

ROUND LAKE TRAIL

GOLF COURSE

GETTING THERE

From I-90 (New York State Thruway), take Exit 34 to I-481 South. Follow I-481 South 1 mile to Kirkville Road exit. Follow Kirkville Road 1 mile to Fremont Road. Turn right on Fremont Road. After 1 mile, turn left on CR 290; follow 3 miles to park entrance on the right.

GPS COORDINATES

PARK ENTRANCE:

UTM Zone (WGS84)   18T
Easting   420897
Northing   4767905
Latitude   N 43°03'35"
Longitude   W 75°58'17"

purchased by the park in the 1980s. Mountain bikers looking for gentle, scenic pedaling would be hard-pressed to find better trails elsewhere. If you do bring your bike, pay attention to signs: a handful of the park's trails are designated for foot traffic only. This includes the wonderfully named Hernia Hill, which only masochists would want to tackle on a bike anyway.

Golf, whether in traditional form or by way of a Frisbee, is available to those who seek it. The 18 holes on the southeast end of the park constitute one of the area's best public courses. And the clubhouse with its outdoor restaurant serves up lovely views of Green Lake to go with burgers and sandwiches. The disc-golf course, found near Pine Wood, is a confidence booster for those of us with laughable golf swings but a great Frisbee toss.

Two of the authors of this book grew up in a house literally yards from the border of Green Lakes State Park and spent their childhoods exploring its 1,756 acres. It is hard to avoid some nostalgia, but we must say that after traveling throughout the state and seeing many wonderful campgrounds and parks, we still keep coming back to visit. Hopefully, after spending a weekend at Green Lakes, you'll do the same.

19
HUNT'S POND STATE PARK

ONE OF THE JOYS OF CAMPING is leaving your world behind. All the campgrounds featured in this book promise an escape from the typical hustle and bustle. Hunt's Pond promises an escape from the typical campground. Some people use camping as a cheap and easy way to access great hikes, trailer boat launches, and tourist attractions. Hunt's Pond cannot compete with other parks in those departments. But for people who consider pitching a tent, building a campfire, and listening to the sounds of nature as vacation enough, there are few better places in the state to spend a night.

Located between Utica and Binghamton a few miles southwest of the town of New Berlin, Hunt's Pond is a nearly one-hour drive from any highway. To the east, the Unadilla River winds its way south until it empties into the Susquehanna. Fly fishermen and paddlers dip into the river's twisting waters on sunny days, thanks in part to the efforts of the Upper Unadilla Valley Association, which opposed plans to flood the valley 30 years ago. Golf courses, nearby parks with beaches, and patches of wild forest distributed throughout the area's farmland provide outdoor recreation for those who seek it. Along the marshy shores of Hunt's Pond itself, you will find a car-top boat launch and rental rowboats, a new picnic pavilion, and 18 primitive camping sites—but little else. Don't worry about cavalcades of RVs and day-trippers here.

The campground rarely fills up and reservations are only necessary if you have a particular site you desire. If you do reserve a site, you should still make sure to register from 4 p.m. to 8 p.m. at the campground office. If you plan to bring a boat (car-top vessels only), register that at the office as well. Because the campground is small and requires less maintenance than most, the staff may not always be present, so be

> *Its marshy, lily pad–lined shores are good for fishing and relaxed paddling.*

RATINGS

Beauty: ✩ ✩ ✩
Privacy: ✩ ✩ ✩ ✩ ✩
Quiet: ✩ ✩ ✩ ✩ ✩
Cleanliness: ✩ ✩ ✩ ✩
Security: ✩ ✩
Spaciousness: ✩ ✩ ✩ ✩

KEY INFORMATION

patient. While you are there, fill up on fresh drinking water from the campground's one spigot. The two comfort stations in the campground consist of pit toilets, but no plumbing. Also, this is a carry-in, carry-out facility, so remember to bring your own trash bags.

The pond's shape vaguely resembles a peanut. As the camp road follows the shoreline, sites 1 through 8 are the first and, in many ways, the best in the campground. All are grassy and with ample shade—and what they may lack in cleared space, they make up for in privacy. For the best views of the pond, site 4 is hard to beat. Perched atop a small incline, site 5 is also a great choice.

On the other side of the pond, sites 9 through 13 are even better spaced, and the fir trees that stretch upward in this loop give it an airy feel. Site 9 is the jewel of the bunch. It is completely isolated and right on the water. A walk of about 30 yards from your car awaits if you choose sites 10 or 12—well worth the effort for the privacy and water views they afford. Avoid site 11—it is right on the campground road and exposed. Site 13 is also open and exposed, but does at least give a great vista of the water.

On the outer reaches of the park, a pine forest forms the border of a grassy field. This is where sites 16 through 18 are found. Unless you are looking to sunbathe or practice your golf putting, there is little reason to choose these wide-open spaces. It would perhaps be a good place for an afternoon barbecue or a game of catch, but for an overnight stay, these are essentially RV or overflow sites. It is unlikely that you have to worry about being forced into this corner of the park.

A gravel road past the office leads to the park's only day-use facilities, consisting of the picnic pavilion, a comfort station, and the car-top boat launch. There is no swimming allowed, and no motorboats are permitted on the water. The surface of Hunt's Pond is approximately 50 acres, and its marshy, lily pad–lined shores are good for fishing and relaxed paddling. The 250-acre park allows hunting in season, but the absence of trails means you will have to travel out of the park for a hike. You will not have to travel far, though.

MAP

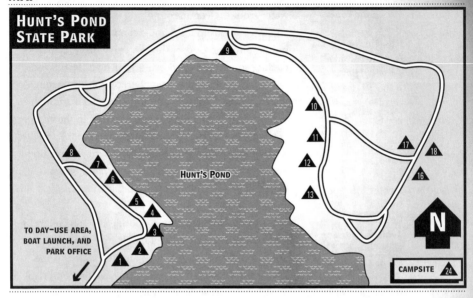

HUNT'S POND STATE PARK

HUNT'S POND

TO DAY-USE AREA, BOAT LAUNCH, AND PARK OFFICE

N

CAMPSITE 24

Surrounding the park is Hunt's Pond State Forest, 1,147 acres of hardwoods, beaver meadows, and softwoods planted by the state when it purchased the land in the 1960s. Unmarked trails wind through European larch, red pine, and Norway spruce. Beavers, deer, and a variety of birds are common sights. Maintained by the Department of Environmental Conservation, the forest is separate from the state park. Backcountry camping is allowed within its borders and will certainly bring hikers extreme solitude (there are restrictions: contact the State Forest office at [607] 674-4036 for details).

Bigger parks with more recreational opportunities are within driving distance, but it hardly seems worth the effort. Beaches and playgrounds and golf courses are a dime a dozen in New York. When campers talk about a weekend of fresh air and peace and quiet, it's nice to know that Hunt's Pond proves there are still a few places where that actually still exists.

GETTING THERE

From I-88, take Exit 9 to NY 8 North. Follow NY 8 for approximately 20 miles to the town of New Berlin. Turn left on Buttermilk Falls Road, then bear right on Hunts Pond Road. Follow Hunts Pond Road for approximately 1.5 miles. Park entrance is on right.

GPS COORDINATES

PARK ENTRANCE:

UTM Zone (WGS84)	18T
Easting	468990
Northing	4715798
Latitude	N 42°35'38"
Longitude	W 75°22'41"

20
MAX V. SHAUL STATE PARK

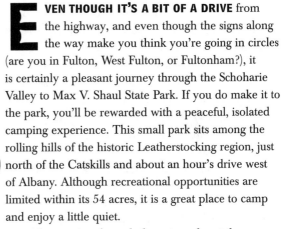

> *Max V. Shaul State Park is a great example of the advantages of a small park with only a handful of campsites.*

EVEN THOUGH IT'S A BIT OF A DRIVE from the highway, and even though the signs along the way make you think you're going in circles (are you in Fulton, West Fulton, or Fultonham?), it is certainly a pleasant journey through the Schoharie Valley to Max V. Shaul State Park. If you do make it to the park, you'll be rewarded with a peaceful, isolated camping experience. This small park sits among the rolling hills of the historic Leatherstocking region, just north of the Catskills and about an hour's drive west of Albany. Although recreational opportunities are limited within its 54 acres, it is a great place to camp and enjoy a little quiet.

After passing through the gate and past the unassuming park office, stay right on the main camp road, and make your way through the hardwoods—lush and green in summer and bursting with reds and yellows in fall. Appropriately, maple-leaf markers designate the 30 nicely shaded sites distributed along two joined loops. A rough paved road winds uphill through the first loop, with sites numbers 1 through 22. Sites on the loop's exterior are the most desirable. They are flat and on the small side, but spacious enough for a tent or two. Set back at least 15 yards from the road and enveloped by thick circles of the trees, sites 3, 4, 13, and 21 stand out as the best. Sites 17 through 20 are close to the road, but are the most widely spaced from each other. Located along the park's outer boundary, they are also bordered by a steep rise to Toe Path Mountain. Site 17 is wheelchair accessible. Water spigots are well placed throughout the loop, and the centrally located comfort station is relatively easy to find in the dark.

Rarely does the park reach capacity, and unless you want a specific site, reservations are recommended only on holiday weekends. None of the sites could be considered bad, but the second loop (sites 23 through

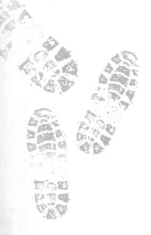

RATINGS

Beauty: ✿ ✿ ✿
Privacy: ✿ ✿ ✿ ✿
Quiet: ✿ ✿ ✿ ✿ ✿
Cleanliness: ✿ ✿ ✿ ✿
Security: ✿ ✿ ✿ ✿
Spaciousness: ✿ ✿ ✿ ✿

30) is certainly the least-private corner of the camp-ground. These spaces are right next to new comfort stations, a swing set, a picnic area, and a series of small parking areas. This may be appealing to families with little ones or to people expecting visitors. A group-camping area opens up behind site 30, where NY 30 meets Panther Creek. If you camp here, you may have a family reunion or perhaps some scouts as neighbors.

This park differs from many state-run campgrounds in that it has no major day-use facilities. Picnicking may attract the occasional family, but the park is primarily used by campers. There is a new basketball hoop, a small playground, a softball diamond, and a horseshoe pit to keep people entertained. In general, this is not a destination that draws campers from many miles away.

Fishing is allowed in Panther Creek across NY 30; just stay along the sections that are inside the park boundary, as much of the creek runs through private property. Outside of Max V. Shaul State Park, there are several other options for anglers. Schoharie Creek runs through the center of the valley and is stocked with brown trout. Looking Glass Pond, an artificial body of water in Fulton, is full of largemouth bass.

A trail starting near site 16 leads out of the campground for a short hike up Toe Path Mountain. Campers arriving from the north may spot another popular local hiking destination known as Vroman's Nose, where the land rises dramatically 600 feet up from the valley floor. The short and steep trail is part of the Long Path, a 335-mile trail running from the New Jersey end of the George Washington Bridge north along the Palisades and through the Shawangunk and Catskill mountains, finally ending at John Boyd Thacher Park outside of Albany. This slice of the path offers great, unobstructed views of the valley.

Nearby attractions include other state parks, historical sites, and caves. Tours of the perennially popular Howe Caverns leave daily and showcase an underground river. Neighboring Howe, the lesser-known Secret Caverns is smaller but contains many oddly shaped formations and a 100-foot underground water-fall that should delight all ages. The cool year-round

KEY INFORMATION

ADDRESS:	Route 30, P.O. Box 23 Fultonham, NY 12071
OPERATED BY:	New York State Office of Parks, Recreation and Historic Preservation
INFORMATION:	(518) 827-4711; nysparks.state.ny.us
OPEN:	Mid-May–early October
SITES:	31
EACH SITE HAS:	Picnic table and fire ring
ASSIGNMENT:	Choose from available sites or reservations
REGISTRATION:	On arrival or by reservation (reserve minimum 2 nights)
FACILITIES:	Water, flush toilets, hot showers, pay phone
PARKING:	At site, maximum 2 vehicles
FEE:	$13/night (plus $3/night for Friday, Saturday, and holidays)
ELEVATION:	708 feet
RESTRICTIONS:	*Pets:* Dogs on leash with proof of cur-rently valid rabies vaccination *Fires:* In fire rings only *Alcohol:* At site *Vehicles:* Up to 30 feet *Other:* Quiet hours 10 p.m.–7 a.m.; carry out all trash *Reservations:* 2-night stay required

MAP

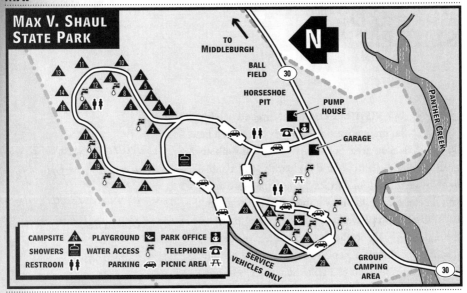

Max V. Shaul State Park

TO MIDDLEBURGH

N

BALL FIELD · 30

HORSESHOE PIT

PUMP HOUSE

GARAGE

PANTHER CREEK

CAMPSITE	▲24	PLAYGROUND		PARK OFFICE	
SHOWERS		WATER ACCESS		TELEPHONE	
RESTROOM		PARKING		PICNIC AREA	⊼

SERVICE VEHICLES ONLY

GROUP CAMPING AREA · 30

GETTING THERE

From I-88, take Exit 22 (Cobleskill/Middleburgh) to NY 145 South. Follow NY 145 for approximately 8 miles to the town of Middleburgh. Turn right on NY 30. Follow NY 30 south for approximately 6 miles. Park entrance is on the right.

GPS COORDINATES

PARK ENTRANCE:

UTM Zone (WGS84)   18T
Easting   548429
Northing   4710621
Latitude   N 42°32'47"
Longitude   W 74°24'37"

underground temperatures of 52°F make both caves great places to visit on a hot summer day.

Another way to cool off is at Mine Kill State Park, where campers can enter free during the length of their stay at Max V. Shaul (be sure to bring your camping receipt). You will need to pay a small fee per person if you plan to use their bathing complex, complete with wading, diving, and Olympic-size swimming pools.

Finally, Cooperstown and the Baseball Hall of Fame (about an hour's drive away) are the centerpieces of the surrounding Leatherstocking region's long and rich history. As for Max V. Shaul State Park, its story is a little more recent. The land was donated by and named after a local farmer and involved citizen, Max V. Shaul. The park opened in 1960 and was rededicated upon Shaul's death in 1980.

Max V. Shaul State Park is a great example of the advantages of a small park with only a handful of campsites. Although there are a number of things to keep campers busy in the area, the real attraction of the campground is the quiet. Even though you may not be pitching your tent in wilderness that stretches for miles, you will still feel that you have the woods to yourself.

21

MOREAU LAKE STATE PARK

MANY VISITORS COME to Moreau Lake for the main attraction—a sandy beach in a land-locked area. Some picnickers and sunbathers even venture out and around the park's Mud Pond to enjoy a nature trail. But stay a night or more and you'll get a chance to know a third body of water in the park—the Hudson River. Carving a winding path through the park's northeast corner, the river passes through breathtaking scenery and by several primitive boat-in campsites. Moreau Lake State Park is techni-cally part of the Adirondack foothills; the "blue line" on maps that marks the border of the Adirondack. Forest Preserve is less than 2 miles to the north. But Moreau is a distinct park on its own, and its clear waters, green woods, and pleasant camping loops are sure to satisfy campers looking for an easily accessible bit of nature.

Moreau Lake is a nearly four-hour drive from Manhattan, but perhaps more importantly, just ten min-utes from the New York Thruway. Visitors intent on get-ting to the beach may never even see the campground. Beyond the park office and registration booth, the camp road splits, leading left to the beach and day-use facili-ties and right to the campground. Pick up ice and fire-wood at the office. There is a $1 deposit for the burlap wood bags, which are an environmentally friendly alter-native to the standard shrink-wrap plastic that so often litters sites. After registering, follow the main road past the wooden guard posts that mark the steep drop to lake's edge. There are seven camping loops to choose from, some bordering each other and some skirting the edge of metal fence that marks the border of the park with Mountain Road. There is just one shower building, located between Loops E and F, but comfort stations are well distributed in the center of each loop.

Mixed hardwoods and firs shade the sites, which will fill-up with an equal mix of RVs, pop-up trailers,

> *Moreau is one of many kettle-hole lakes formed by glaciers carving out the land.*

RATINGS

Beauty: ☆ ☆ ☆
Privacy: ☆ ☆ ☆
Quiet: ☆ ☆ ☆
Cleanliness: ☆ ☆ ☆
Security: ☆ ☆ ☆ ☆
Spaciousness: ☆ ☆ ☆

ADDRESS:	605 Old Saratoga Road Gansevoort, NY 12831
OPERATED BY:	New York State Office of Parks, Recreation and Historic Preservation
INFORMATION:	(518) 793-0511; nysparks.state.ny.us
OPEN:	Mid-May–early October
SITES:	148 plus 2 boat-in sites
EACH SITE HAS:	Picnic table and fire ring
ASSIGNMENT:	Choose from available sites or reservations
REGISTRATION:	On arrival or by reservation (reserve minimum 2 nights)
FACILITIES:	Water, flush toilets, showers, pay phone
PARKING:	At site, maximum 2 vehicles
FEE:	$13/night (plus $3/night on Friday, Saturday, and holidays)
ELEVATION:	215 feet
RESTRICTIONS:	*Pets:* Dogs on leash with proof of currently valid rabies vaccination *Fires:* In fire rings only *Alcohol:* At site *Vehicles:* Up to 40 feet *Other:* Quiet hours 10 p.m.–7 a.m.; no motorboats *Reservations:* 2-night stay required

and tents. Reservations are a necessity during summer weekends. Loop A features flat, roomy, nicely wooded spaces, and was the least crowded when we visited. Loop B is smaller, with some of the most well-spaced sites, but houses can be seen through the trees, especially when the trees lose their leaves, spoiling the illusion of being deep in the woods. Loops C and D are on rough roads up a steep hill from the lake, with spotty views of the water through the trees. Some campers reserve these sites, mistakenly thinking they are getting prime lakefront spots, but they are a nice option nonetheless. Site 72 in Loop D has grown to be one of the largest, evidence that equipment set on the edge of the site reduces the surrounding vegetation over time. Loops F and G are well removed from the rest, but the sites are more congested—and again, views of a nearby residential development can be an annoyance.

To really get away from it all, bring a sturdy boat and access one of the two primitive boat-in sites on the Hudson. Bennie Brook and the deceptively named Sherman Island (actually near, not on an island) are such nice places to camp that the park plans to develop several more riverside sites in the future. The sites are little more than a fire-ring in a clearing—sorry, no picnic tables or toilets here. Reservations are not available and they fill up on a first-come, first-served basis. But it is not a matter of making a mad dash down the river. Campers must first obtain a free overnight-parking pass from the campground office and use one of the two boat ramps on Spier Falls Road to access the river from inside the park.

The park has built a causeway footbridge to separate the two sections of the semicolon-shaped lake. Moreau is one of many kettle-hole lakes formed by glaciers carving out the land. Past the park's lone rental cottage is the beach complex, with parking, designated swimming area, store, snack bar, and nature center, which hosts daily events in summer. Whether you want to rent fishing poles and tackle or umbrellas and lounge chairs, you can find them here. No motorboats are allowed on the lake, but this is not necessarily the quietest corner of the park—the beach gets very busy on warm days.

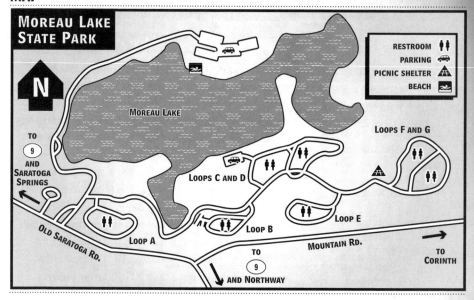

MOREAU LAKE STATE PARK

RESTROOM	♀♂
PARKING	🚗
PICNIC SHELTER	⛺
BEACH	🏊

MOREAU LAKE

TO 9 AND SARATOGA SPRINGS

LOOPS F AND G

LOOPS C AND D

OLD SARATOGA RD.

LOOP A

LOOP B

LOOP E

MOUNTAIN RD.

TO CORINTH

TO 9 AND NORTHWAY

More than 20 miles of trails crisscross the Palmertown Mountain Range, a series of 1,000-foot bumps that border the southern side of the Hudson. All 12 trails are clearly marked, but we recommend picking up a topographic map at the park office—well worth the $2 fee. These are multiuse trails, so watch out for mountain bikes. Trails range in distance, starting with the steep but short Overlook Trail and its great views of the lake. The Nature Trail is just over 1 mile, with an interpretive loop that runs over the causeway, through Loop D, and reaches Mud Pond. Another option is the Western Ridge Trail, which climbs 5 miles to Spring Overlook. Enjoy the view of the Northern Luzerne Mountain Range across the bend in the river and keep an eye out for hawks and eagles.

Lake Moreau is a great place to stay while exploring the surrounding area. Twenty miles to the north is Lake George, with its many recreational activities; 10 miles to the south are the famed horse tracks of Saratoga Springs. Thankfully, campers can avoid the Lake George crowds and will not be gambling by pitching a tent at Moreau Lake.

GETTING THERE

From I-87 (Adirondack Northway), take Exit 17S, South Glen Falls, to NY 9 South. Take first right on Old Saratoga Road. Drive less than 1 mile to park entrance on right.

GPS COORDINATES

PARK ENTRANCE:

UTM Zone (WGS84)   18T
Easting   605034
Northing   4787165
Latitude   N 43°13'48"
Longitude   W 73°42'24"

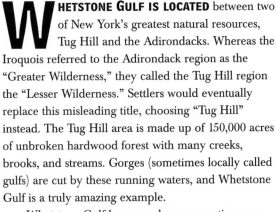

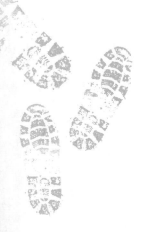

> *Explore the "Lesser Wilderness" while camping at the outlet of a 3-mile gorge.*

WHETSTONE **GULF IS LOCATED** between two of New York's greatest natural resources, Tug Hill and the Adirondacks. Whereas the Iroquois referred to the Adirondack region as the "Greater Wilderness," they called the Tug Hill region the "Lesser Wilderness." Settlers would eventually replace this misleading title, choosing "Tug Hill" instead. The Tug Hill area is made up of 150,000 acres of unbroken hardwood forest with many creeks, brooks, and streams. Gorges (sometimes locally called gulfs) are cut by these running waters, and Whetstone Gulf is a truly amazing example.

Whetstone Gulf has served as a recreation area since the 1800s and was formally acquired as a state park in the 1920s. Improvements by the New York State Conservation Department and the Civilian Conservation Corps followed during the 1930s and again after WWII. Evidence of their hard work can be seen today, including a man-made beach, bridges, trails, and plantings of red pine, a fast-growing species seen throughout the park.

Of the 62 campsites, 56 are situated among these tall pines, which provide plenty of shade and a bit of privacy from neighboring sites. The spacious sites are located along several one-way loops. Three comfort stations and one shower serve the area. Water spigots and multiple dumpsters with recycling are located along the loops. Sites along the north edge of the campground are screened from the main park road by dense pines and understory brush. Most interior sites are openly visible to each other, and though they provide less privacy than those along the edge, the dense trees give the area an atmosphere of a woodland rather than an open campground. Sites along the east and south edges are more secluded, private, and spacious. The southern sites are farther apart and benefit

RATINGS

Beauty: ✪ ✪
Privacy: ✪ ✪ ✪
Quiet: ✪ ✪ ✪
Cleanliness: ✪ ✪ ✪
Security: ✪ ✪
Spaciousness: ✪ ✪ ✪

from a dense understory that has begun to grow as the native hardwood forest encroaches. Each site has a stone fire pit with grill top, gravel drive, and adequate space for spreading out. The 12 sites with electric hookups are primarily located in the interior.

Situated off the parking area near the beach and Whetstone Creek, the last six sites are essentially overflow sites. These sites are wide open, directly next to each other, and adjacent to much of park's foot traffic and other activities. Reservations are recommended for weekends and holidays, as most sites are booked well in advance. Weekday campers can expect available sites without reservations.

The park's swimming area, created by the damming of Whetstone Creek, is only a short walk from the main campsite area. You can reach a playground, bathhouse, and a recreation building directly from the beach. Past the beach and across a short bridge is the park's picnic area, accessed along a road that follows Whetstone Creek up the gorge. There are plenty of picnic tables and charcoal grills along this meandering road, but the wooded views of the gulf at this point are mere temptations, as the gorge's most dramatic views are accessible only to the hiker.

A 5-mile loop trail encircles much of the 3-mile gulf. Be aware that the trail lies directly along the gorge rim, and that the path is strewn with exposed tree roots, so take care at all times. Hikers can begin their trek on either the north or south rim. To obtain the best views, which are only accessible where the trails meet on the gorge's western end, plan to complete the entire circuit. The only significant difference between the two trails is that the South Rim Trail has a watch tower that offers views to the east. On the eastern segment of the trails, the gorge's sides are steep but heavily vegetated. Consequently, views across the gulf offer only brief glimpses of the drastic erosion that has taken place. As hikers move west, the gorge narrows, the sides become more sheer, and the vegetation thins to reveal exposed shale. At the western end, the gulf's 385-foot walls are vertical and fully exposed. Campers visiting the park shouldn't miss these dramatic views.

KEY INFORMATION

ADDRESS:	6065 West Road Lowville, NY 13367
OPERATED BY:	New York State Office of Parks, Recreation and Historic Preservation
INFORMATION:	(315) 376-6630; nysparks.state.ny.us
OPEN:	Memorial Day–mid-September
SITES:	62 tent sites, 12 electric sites
EACH SITE HAS:	Stone fire pit, picnic table
ASSIGNMENT:	Choose from available sites or reservations
REGISTRATION:	3 p.m.–9 p.m.
FACILITIES:	Picnic tables, bathhouse, pavilion, potable water, flush toilets, showers
PARKING:	At site
FEE:	$13/night
ELEVATION:	1,300 feet
RESTRICTIONS:	*Pets:* Dogs on leash with proof of currently valid rabies vaccination *Fires:* In fire pits only *Alcohol:* Allowed *Vehicles:* RVs and trailers allowed *Other:* Quiet hours 10 p.m.–7 a.m. *Reservations:* 2-night stay required; 6 people maximum/site; maximum 14-night stay

MAP

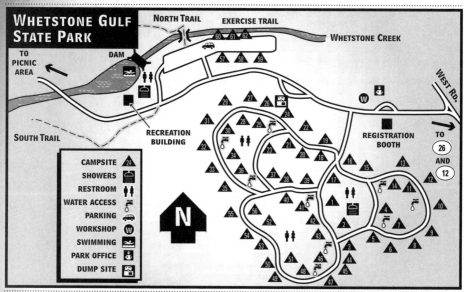

WHETSTONE GULF STATE PARK

NORTH TRAIL
EXERCISE TRAIL
WHETSTONE CREEK
TO PICNIC AREA
DAM
SOUTH TRAIL
RECREATION BUILDING
REGISTRATION BOOTH
WEST RD.
TO
AND

CAMPSITE	
SHOWERS	
RESTROOM	
WATER ACCESS	
PARKING	
WORKSHOP	
SWIMMING	
PARK OFFICE	
DUMP SITE	

GETTING THERE

From I-87 (New York State Thruway), take Exit 31, NY 8/NY 12. After toll, turn right on Genesee Street toward I-790 West/NY 5. Turn right on Aubert Avenue and merge onto I-790 West/NY 5 toward NY 12/NY 8. Merge onto NY 12 North toward Poland/Watertown; follow 29.5 miles. Park entrance is on right.

GPS COORDINATES

PARK ENTRANCE:
UTM Zone (WGS84)   18T
Easting   462923
Northing   4838943
Latitude   N 43°42'09"
Longitude   W 75°72'37"

Other activities within the park's boundaries include an exercise trail, as well as fishing and canoeing in the Whetstone Gulf Reservoir. The reservoir was constructed to provide flood control of Whetstone Creek as well as recreational opportunities. The reservoir is accessible from Corrigan Hill Road and is stocked with tiger muskies and largemouth bass.

Hikers wanting more-extensive trails can also visit the Lesser Wilderness State Forest, which borders much of Whetstone Gulf State Park. Whetstone's 2,100 acres combined with Lesser Wilderness's 13,793 makes an extensive, continuous wilderness area. Hiking the access roads and trails and fishing the streams and brooks expand the outdoor recreational activities directly accessible from the park.

The Tug Hill area has many state forests, preserves, recreation areas, and wildlife management areas that provide hiking, bicycling, fishing, canoeing, and kayaking opportunities—so travelers may want to consider this campground as a base camp to explore other points of interest in the "Lesser Wilderness."

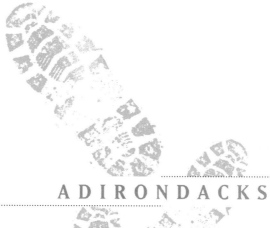

ADIRONDACKS

THIS SCENIC CAMPGROUND is located at the western end of Fourth Lake, a central part of the Fulton Chain of lakes. The Fulton Chain is a series of connected lakes that begins at Old Forge Pond and ends at Eighth Lake. The first five lakes stretch unbroken for 14 miles. Old Forge Pond and Sixth through Eighth lakes are separated from this main expanse by a series of channels. Steamboat inventor Robert Fulton envisioned connecting the lakes and creating an "Adirondack Canal." Although the canal was never built, the lakes still bear Fulton's name.

The lakes were eventually dammed and connected to provide flood control, recreational opportunities, and power in Lyons Falls. The shores are dotted with numerous summer "camps," or private residences, and boathouses—not mere storage buildings for boats, but actual homes ranging from quaint cottages to luxurious estates dating back to the Gilded Age. Though the shoreline is certainly developed, the area is heavily wooded. Views from the lakes reveal rocky outcroppings and a vast, serene wilderness that have drawn outdoors enthusiasts to this region for generations.

First known as Deer Island, then Big Island, the name eventually changed to Alger Island after its longtime owners Mort and Ollie Alger. The state acquired the island in 1950 and began to build lean-tos in the 1960s. Each site is heavily wooded with evergreens and situated a stone's throw from the water's edge. Sites along the northern shore face the lakes' main channel, so boat tours, waterskiers, and Jet Skis are occasional disturbances during the day. A charming lighthouse is also visible from the northern shore. Sites on the southern shore border a small inlet and provide more seclusion. Access is limited to registered campers, and isolation from the mainland ensures privacy and security.

> *Enjoy private lakeside camping in the heart of the Adirondacks.*

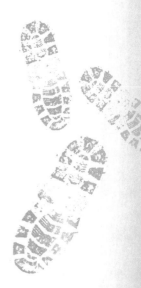

RATINGS

Beauty: ☆ ☆ ☆ ☆
Privacy: ☆ ☆ ☆ ☆
Quiet: ☆ ☆ ☆
Cleanliness: ☆ ☆ ☆ ☆
Security: ☆ ☆ ☆ ☆ ☆
Spaciousness: ☆ ☆ ☆

ADDRESS: P.O. Box 347, CR 18 Old Forge NY, 13420

OPERATED BY: New York State Department of Environmental Conservation

INFORMATION: (315) 369-3224; www.dec.state.ny.us/website/do/camping

OPEN: Mid-May–early September

SITES: 15 lean-to sites, 2 tent sites

EACH SITE HAS: Lean-to (except the 2 tent sites), pit toilet, and fire ring

ASSIGNMENT: Reservations

REGISTRATION: 12 p.m.–9 p.m.; required for access to island

FACILITIES: Picnic area, potable water, docks, lean-tos

PARKING: At Fourth Lake picnic area

FEE: $14/night

ELEVATION: 520 feet

RESTRICTIONS: 6 people maximum/site, maximum 14-night stay, access only by boat
Pets: Dogs on leash with proof of currently valid rabies vaccination
Fires: In fire rings only
Alcohol: Allowed
Vehicles: Vehicles park at Fourth Lake Picnic Area
Other: Quiet hours 10 p.m.–7 a.m.
Reservations: None required for the 2 tent sites, required for lean-tos; 2-night stay required

Campers should be aware that the only way to get to the island is by boat. A state-owned boat launch is located at the Fourth Lake picnic area. This picnic area also serves as the Alger Island registration and permitting station. Boats launched at this facility are limited to car-top boats such as kayaks; motorboats can be launched from the public launch in Inlet. For campers who don't own boats, numerous outfitters along NY 28 not only rent boats but also offer rafting packages. The popularity of this campground is evident; most sites are fully booked during July and August, with the most popular sites being booked a year in advance.

Hiking at the campground is limited to a perimeter trail, but access to the central region of the Adirondacks provides miles of hiking opportunities. Hiking terrain in the region is generally hilly and rugged but not mountainous. Most of the surrounding area is heavily forested and within the protected Forest Preserve Area of the Adirondack State Park. Trails are often old logging roads that have become overgrown as they transform back into wilderness. Large, expansive views are limited, but numerous lakes, ponds, swamps, and streams present surprises around every corner. Most trails are can be done as day hikes and can be reached from NY 12 and NY 28.

Fishing is permitted at the campground and on the lake with a New York state fishing license. Smallmouth bass, lake trout, brook trout, rainbow trout, and land-locked Atlantic salmon are found in Fourth Lake, and muskie and largemouth bass can be caught in some of the adjoining Fulton Chain of lakes. Swimming is allowed in the lake but there is no designated swimming area; swimmers should be mindful of boating activities nearby. A sandbar on the north shore near site 6 offers the best swimming area. Motorboats, canoes, and rowboats can be tied up at the docks on the southern or eastern shores; this allows campers to participate in a variety of Fulton Chain boating activities.

Considered the main tourist destination of the central region, the town of Old Forge offers many attractions for those interested in local history and entertainment. Of note are the renovated theatre, Water Park, Old Forge Hardware Store, and the

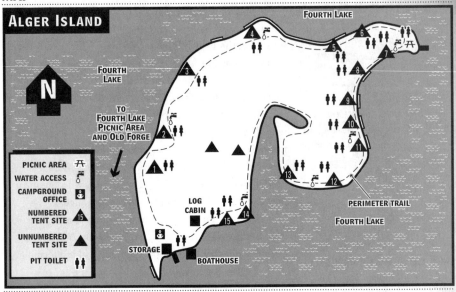

ALGER ISLAND

FOURTH LAKE

FOURTH LAKE

TO
FOURTH LAKE
PICNIC AREA
AND OLD FORGE

PERIMETER TRAIL

FOURTH LAKE

LOG
CABIN

STORAGE

BOATHOUSE

PICNIC AREA	🜨
WATER ACCESS	🚰
CAMPGROUND OFFICE	🏢
NUMBERED TENT SITE	▲15
UNNUMBERED TENT SITE	▲
PIT TOILET	👫

Adirondack Scenic Railroad. Supplies and equipment can be purchased along NY 28 from numerous outfitters, and also in small grocery stores in Old Forge, Eagle Bay, or Inlet.

Alger Island Campground's rocky shores and evergreen canopy provide a unique lakeside camping experience in one of New York's most cherished parks and wilderness areas. Outdoor activities abound in the region, and proximity to Old Forge allows campers to easily stock up on supplies and equipment.

GETTING THERE

Use directions on page 83 through fourth sentence, but
take NY 12 North 22.3 miles. Bear right onto NY 28 North; go 26.7 miles to Old Forge. Go right on Gilbert Street, left on Park Avenue, then right on South Shore Road. After 5.9 miles, make a sharp left onto Petrie Road. Fourth Lake Picnic Area is 0.75 miles on left.

GPS COORDINATES

ALGER ISLAND:

UTM Zone (WGS84)	18T
Easting	509908
Northing	4843281
Latitude	N 43°44'33"
Longitude	W 74°52'37"

GPS COORDINATES

FOURTH LAKE PICNIC AREA:

UTM Zone (WGS84)	18T
Easting	508724
Northing	4842539
Latitude	N 43°44'09"
Longitude	W 74°53'30"

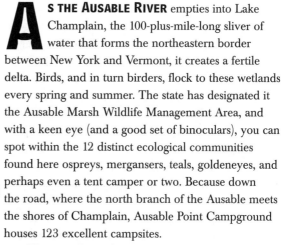

> *For a relatively young campground (built in 1965), Ausable Point sits on the shores of a body of water with a long history.*

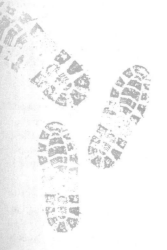

AS THE **AUSABLE RIVER** empties into Lake Champlain, the 100-plus-mile-long sliver of water that forms the northeastern border between New York and Vermont, it creates a fertile delta. Birds, and in turn birders, flock to these wetlands every spring and summer. The state has designated it the Ausable Marsh Wildlife Management Area, and with a keen eye (and a good set of binoculars), you can spot within the 12 distinct ecological communities found here ospreys, mergansers, teals, goldeneyes, and perhaps even a tent camper or two. Because down the road, where the north branch of the Ausable meets the shores of Champlain, Ausable Point Campground houses 123 excellent campsites.

The campground entrance road leads along the northern border of Ausable Marsh. Even if you're not a birder, pull over and read the interpretive signs, or look out over the water from a viewing dock. A mile-long elevated foot trail will bring you closer to some of the ecological communities, including emergent marsh, floodplain forest, and marsh headwater stream. If you are indeed a birder, the Lake Champlain Birding Trail site (**www.lakechamplainbirding.org**) is an excellent resource to consult beforehand.

At the end of the road, just past the registration booth, is the campground's gem of a beach. More than a quarter-mile of sand makes up the large day-use area, complete with a new pavilion and bathhouse. Lifeguards regularly oversee the designated swimming areas. The size of the parking area testifies to the number of day visitors that use the beach and picnic area. Be prepared to share. The silver lining: there are no vendors hawking pizza and fried food, and that helps keep some folks away. East of the beach is a separate windsurfing area known as the Stone Jetty. If the crowds at the swimming beach are a bit too oppressive,

RATINGS

Beauty: ☆ ☆ ☆
Privacy: ☆ ☆
Quiet: ☆ ☆ ☆
Cleanliness: ☆ ☆ ☆
Security: ☆ ☆ ☆
Spaciousness: ☆ ☆ ☆

drop your beach chair near the jetty and enjoy the sight of windsurfers and boaters gliding along Lake Champlain's waters, with Valcour Island as a backdrop.

Just south of Stone Jetty, the relatively private, grass-and-sand campsites are great for pitching a tent. They are laid out in four separate loops, each with its own comfort station and multiple sources of running water. Sites 1 through 24 are closest to the jetty— and with the windsurfer loading area, the camp's new shower building, and a swing set all nearby, this loop tends to be the noisiest during the day. But it also contains the most sites on the edge of Lake Champlain, including 9, 10, 11, 13, 15, 16, 19, 20, 21, and 22. These sites, separated by privacy hedges, are usually booked far in advance. However, we found the second loop (25 through 48) just as desirable. Sites on the eastern perimeter of the loop border a small, grassy marsh. The North Branch of the Ausable skirts the edge of the southern sites. The spacious site 27 was a favorite, ideal for a larger group. Site 28 is sandy and opens onto a small beach—but don't forget that wading and swimming are allowed only at the lifeguard beach.

If you are looking for less through-traffic, consider sites 49 through 80, but be warned that the foliage in this section does not provide as much privacy as one would hope. A small path between sites 77 and 78 takes you directly to the beach, and this may appeal to families with little ones.

Sites 1E through 43E used to be the favorites for RVs, but not anymore. They pulled the plug on these former electric sites in the winter of 2006 because of safety concerns and requirements to keep Adirondack campgrounds rustic. This change has certainly lowered the number of RVs visiting the campground and short-ened the length of some visits, but generators can still be heard during designated hours. For now, the hookup posts remain, reminding campers what they are miss-ing, for better or worse. Try to avoid these sites in the spring or after a storm. With the Ausable running nearby, this section of the campground tends to flood.

Lake Champlain's wide waters are suitable for boats of all types. Paddling is best close to shore and the only launch in the campground is for car-top boats.

KEY INFORMATION

ADDRESS:	3346 Lake Shore Road Peru, NY 12972
OPERATED BY:	New York State Department of Environmental Conservation
INFORMATION:	(518) 561-7080; www.dec.state.ny.us/website/do/camping
OPEN:	Mid-May–early October
SITES:	123
EACH SITE HAS:	Picnic table and fire ring
ASSIGNMENT:	Choose from available sites or reservations
REGISTRATION:	On arrival or by reservation (reserve minimum 2 nights)
FACILITIES:	Water, flush toilets, showers, pay phone
PARKING:	At site; maximum 2 vehicles
FEE:	$18/night
ELEVATION:	98 feet
RESTRICTIONS:	*Pets:* Dogs on leash with proof of cur-rently valid rabies vaccination *Fires:* In fire rings only *Alcohol:* At site *Vehicles:* Up to 45 feet *Other:* Quiet hours 10 p.m.–7 a.m. *Reservations:* 2-night stay required

MAP

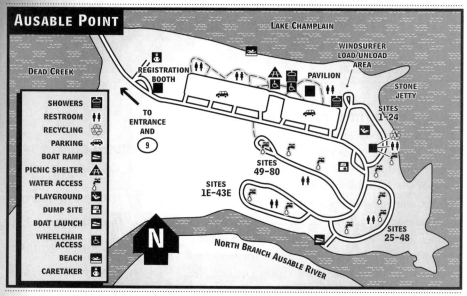

AUSABLE POINT

LAKE CHAMPLAIN

WINDSURFER LOAD/UNLOAD AREA

DEAD CREEK

REGISTRATION BOOTH

PAVILION

STONE JETTY

SITES 1-24

TO ENTRANCE AND

9

SHOWERS
RESTROOM
RECYCLING
PARKING
BOAT RAMP
PICNIC SHELTER
WATER ACCESS
PLAYGROUND
DUMP SITE
BOAT LAUNCH
WHEELCHAIR ACCESS
BEACH
CARETAKER

SITES 49-80

SITES 1E-43E

SITES 25-48

N

NORTH BRANCH AUSABLE RIVER

GETTING THERE

From Interstate 87 (Adirondack Northway), take Exit 35 to CR 442. Follow CR 442 for 2 miles. Turn left on NY 9 North. Drive 0.5 miles to campground entrance on the right.

GPS COORDINATES

PARK ENTRANCE:

UTM Zone (WGS84) 18T
Easting 623726
Northing 4937453
Latitude N 44°34'47"
Longitude W 73°26'29"

A public trailer launch is located 3 miles away at the Peru Docks. Anglers try to catch bass, trout, salmon, bullhead perch, walleye, carp, smelt, eel, crappie, or bluegill from boats or the shore.

Minutes from the campground, the Ausable River thunders through a narrow gorge for 2 miles, forming Ausable Chasm. Sometimes called "Little Grand Canyon of the East," this is not to be confused with the "Grand Canyon of the East" in Letchworth State Park (see page 172). Day-trippers can use the free parking lot, walk over the chasm bridge, and take in the spectacular waterfall and the churning waters that stand in stark contrast to the placid delta where the river empties into Lake Champlain.

For a relatively young campground (built in 1965), Ausable Point sits on the shores of a body of water with a long history. Lake Champlain was named after the French explorer Samuel de Champlain, who first sailed these waters in 1609. For a great tribute to Champlain, check out Crown Point, about an hour's drive to the south. Historic forts and the Champlain Memorial Lighthouse make it worth a stop.

BROWN TRACT POND

MOST VISITORS TO THE Adirondacks think of placid bodies of water whose forested and boulder-strewn shores embody the images of the tranquil wilderness. During the tourist season, campers who seek these settings usually have to hike or boat to primitive campsites—but the Brown Tract Pond campground offers such opportunities for the car camper. Tucked away from the main tourist areas of the Adirondack Park is the 146-acre Brown Tract Pond, whose rugged shores offer tent campers a quiet wilderness setting. Power boats are not allowed on the pond—and given the remote setting, the loudest sounds you are likely to hear will be the calls of a loon.

The campground consists of three separate areas—one neighboring the entrance, one past the day-use area, and one along Uncas Road. The first area includes sites 1 through 37, though the numbering does not follow the direction of travel through the area. The first few grassy sites (30 through 32) are relatively open, with some shade provided by evergreens that obscure views of the pond. As you drive up a small hill, the canopy of evergreens closes, shading the area more thoroughly. Clustered together along the hill are sites 22 through 29, all of which lie on the pond side of the road and have views of the water. Campers should note that sites 23 and 26 are walk-in sites, but because they are directly on the shore, they are very desirable. Across the road and near the area's comfort station are sites 20 and 21, which are similar to the previous sites but lack views of the pond. Atop the hill, undergrowth is notably absent due to the thickening of a evergreen canopy, but campers who prefer views over privacy would be well suited to the pond side of the road, as the views here are expansive. Across the road, the sites begin to blend into the mixed-hardwood forest, offering some privacy at the expense of views

> *Tucked away from the main tourist areas of Adirondack Park is the 146-acre Brown Tract Pond, whose rugged shores offer tent campers a quiet wilderness setting.*

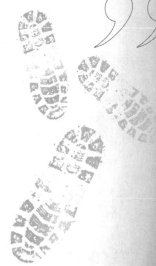

RATINGS

Beauty: ✮ ✮ ✮ ✮ ✮
Privacy: ✮ ✮ ✮ ✮
Quiet: ✮ ✮ ✮ ✮ ✮
Cleanliness: ✮ ✮ ✮ ✮
Security: ✮ ✮ ✮ ✮
Spaciousness: ✮ ✮ ✮

ADDRESS: Uncas Road
Raquette Lake, NY
13436

OPERATED BY: New York State
Department of
Environmental
Conservation

INFORMATION: (315) 354-4412;
www.dec.state.ny.us/
website/do/camping

OPEN: Mid-May–Labor Day

SITES: 90 tent sites

EACH SITE HAS: Picnic table and
fire ring

ASSIGNMENT: Choose from
available sites or
reservations

REGISTRATION: 12 p.m.–9 p.m.

FACILITIES: Picnic areas, potable
water, flush toilets,
boat launch, showers

PARKING: At site

FEE: $14/night; add $3/
night Friday, Satur-
day, and holidays)

ELEVATION: 1,788 feet

RESTRICTIONS: *Pets:* Dogs on leash
with proof of cur-
rently valid rabies
vaccination
Fires: In fire rings
only
Alcohol: Allowed
Vehicles: RVs and
trailers allowed
Other: Quiet hours
10 p.m.–7 a.m.;
6 people maximum/
site; maximum
14-night stay
Reservations: 2-night
stay required

of the pond. The one-way route out of the area dips down into a small hollow that contains sites 1 through 6. Shaded by hardwoods and surrounded by vegetation, these sites feel more private but none have views of the water and all are smaller than previous sites. The last few sites (33 through 37) in the area lie on a separate road next to the pond and are surrounded by thick brush. Though tall shade trees are notably absent from this area, these sites are deep and private. Given the beautiful views of the pond, these sites are definitely among the top choices.

The next camping area is past an evergreen swamp and the public picnic area. The first few sites (38, 48, and 49) sit at a crossroads and are consequently fairly public. The road forks at this point: right is a steep climb to sites 50 through 81; left is to the boat launch and sites 39 through 47. Sites on the left fork hug the pond's shore (except for site 41), and all have excellent views of the water. Short hardwoods provide intermittent shade, but there is little vegetation in the area to provide real seclusion.

As you bear right and drive up the steep hill, the character of the campground changes, as tall hardwoods predominate and a dense woodland feel pervades the area. Sites 50 and 51 along the steep climb are very deep, large, and spacious. Atop the hill are two large, grassy, open sites (52 and 53), after which the road forks to form a loop. Near this fork are short driveways for the walk-in sites (55, 56, and 58) that are situated among rugged woodlands— this creates a very remote feel but leaves little room to spread out. The central sites and upper part of the loop are generally encircled by a dense understory, which creates smaller but isolated sites. At the back of the loop, a short spur road gives access to some larger and more desirable sites (68 through 70). Sites 69 and 70 are walk-in sites, and because they sit high above the water, they have breathtaking views of the pond and the surrounding wilderness. The dense woodland and rugged terrain create wonderfully secluded sites at this point. The next four sites (71 through 74) share access, and although 73 is a secluded walk-in site similar to 69 and 70, the other sites in this group huddle around a

MAP

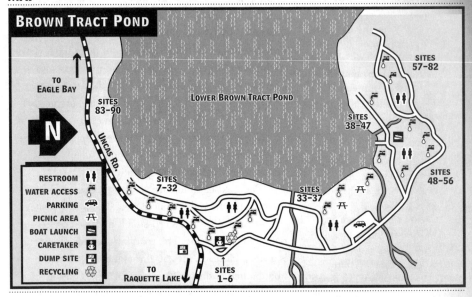

BROWN TRACT POND

TO EAGLE BAY

LOWER BROWN TRACT POND

SITES 57–82

SITES 83–90

UNCAS RD.

SITES 38–47

SITES 48–56

SITES 7–32

SITES 33–37

RESTROOM	
WATER ACCESS	
PARKING	
PICNIC AREA	
BOAT LAUNCH	
CARETAKER	
DUMP SITE	
RECYCLING	

TO RAQUETTE LAKE

SITES 1–6

sandy drive. The rest of the sites along the perimeter of this loop are secluded and well forested, with good views of the pond. The last three (80 through 82) are short walk-ins down the hill; these woodland sites afford plenty of privacy.

Access to the final camping area is directly off Uncas Road; consequently, sites here are removed from the rest of the campground. The large and spacious sites are heavily wooded and offer great views of the pond. The area does not have a comfort station but rather is served by pit toilets. Their proximity to a public dirt road may raise security issues for some campers, but considering the remote location of the campground and the lack of traffic on the bumpy road, this issue is easily overlooked. Indeed, these sites are the first to fill up, and because they offer a private lakeside setting, it is certainly worth taking a look to see what is available.

GETTING THERE

Use directions on page 88 through first sentence. Bear right onto NY 28 North; go past Old Forge and Inlet to Raquette Lake Village. Turn left on CR 2; go 0.5 miles past general store (CR 2 becomes Antlers Road). After 0.2 miles, go left on Uncas Road. Campground entrance is 1.8 miles ahead on right.

GPS COORDINATES

PARK ENTRANCE:

UTM Zone (WGS84) 18T

Easting 524554

Northing 4850862

Latitude N 43°48'38"

Longitude W 74°41'41"

> *Buck Pond is a haven for paddlers.*

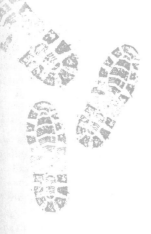

MORE THAN **20** MILES NORTH of Lake Placid and 6 miles from the closest store for supplies, Buck Pond is a truly remote campground and one of our favorites in the Adirondacks. Visitors to the region, including many Canadians (drive 50 miles north and you will be in Quebec), do not come here to find antiques or stay at scenic inns. They come for the woods and the water, and Buck Pond is a haven for paddlers.

Situated between Buck Pond on the east, Kushaqua Narrows on the west, and Lake Kushaqua on the north, the campground is bordered by water. During the summer, most campers (a mix of RVs, pop-ups, and tents) are likely to have at least one boat with them. If you cannot bring your own, there are canoes and rowboats to rent and local outfitters to load you up with gear.

Regulations vary on each body of water. No motorboats are allowed on Buck Pond, guaranteeing a quieter scene. Campers slide their canoes and kayaks into the water from the car-top boat launch (the dock is old—watch out for splinters). Lake Kushaqua and its trailer boat launch offer opportunities for larger (and faster) vessels. Paddlers can travel 7 continuous miles in the water, or more than 100 miles to Old Forge if they don't mind a handful of portages. Less ambitious? If you can carry your boat three-quarters of a mile, a float to the village of Paul Smiths (about 10 miles away by car) is possible. Canoeists and kayakers alike enjoy this trip through the Kushaqua Narrows, Rainbow Lake, Jones Pond, and Osgood Pond. Just plan ahead and, as the campground brochure suggests, have a car waiting at the other end. Or continue south from Paul Smiths to Saranac Lakes, or west into the "forever wild" waters of the St. Regis Canoe Area.

Anglers enjoy a visit to the campground as well, pulling up brown bullhead, northern pike, and yellow

RATINGS

Beauty: ✫ ✫ ✫ ✫
Privacy: ✫ ✫ ✫ ✫
Quiet: ✫ ✫ ✫ ✫
Cleanliness: ✫ ✫ ✫ ✫
Security: ✫ ✫ ✫ ✫
Spaciousness: ✫ ✫ ✫ ✫

perch from Buck Pond and black bass and rainbow trout from Lake Kushaqua. Up the road near Mud Pond, the North Branch of the Saranac River is a good place to find brook trout. If you are turned off by the name Mud Pond, let it be known that there are countless bodies of water in the Adirondacks with this uninviting moniker. As the story goes, some of the best fishing spots are near or on "Mud Ponds," and they were so named to dissuade those not in the know.

Come to think of it, "Buck Pond" isn't the nicest of names, but the campground is certainly a fine one. Driving along the camp road (formerly the route of the Delaware & Hudson rail bed), you may notice the subtle design details that increase one's sense of privacy. The sites are thick with mixed hardwoods and a full understory that shelters campers from their neighbors and the sun. But the angled entrances and staggered sites make the biggest difference. Views of campers from one site to another are rare. If only more campgrounds were this well planned. Another nice touch: each comfort station includes one shower, so there's no need for a long walk (or drive) to a common bathhouse.

Loops A and B curl off to the right just past the registration booth. Sites in Loop A fill up quickly, especially those nearest the water (9, 12, 13, 15, 17, 19, 20, and 21). Along the edge of the campground in Loop B, site 56 is a good choice for those who want even more privacy. Loop C, a double loop with rougher roads, includes some of the sites closest to Lake Kushaqua (most notably sites 89, 91, 92, and 94). It's hard to go wrong with any sites in the campground, though. Even the seven sites in tiny Loop D, near the recycling center, are well spread out.

By far, the most desired are two boat-access sites that are usually booked solid months in advance. A literal stone's throw across the water from 91 and 92, sites I-1 and I-2 sit on a small island and feature the standard fire ring and picnic table, along with pit toilets. Campers could probably wade over to the island, but it is still a nice thought to be sharing your land with just one other group. Even if you do not get an island site, relax at the sandy bathing beach

KEY INFORMATION

ADDRESS:	CR 60 P.O. Box 9A Onchiota, NY
OPERATED BY:	New York State Department of Environmental Conservation
INFORMATION:	(518) 891-3449; www.dec.state.ny.us/website/do/camping
OPEN:	Mid-May–early September
SITES:	116
EACH SITE HAS:	Picnic table and fire ring
ASSIGNMENT:	Choose from available sites or reservations
REGISTRATION:	On arrival or by reservation (reserve minimum 2 nights)
FACILITIES:	Water, pit and flush toilets, showers, pay phone
PARKING:	At site, maximum 2 vehicles
FEE:	$16/night
ELEVATION:	1,696 feet
RESTRICTIONS:	*Pets:* Dogs on leash with proof of currently valid rabies vaccination *Fires:* In fire rings only *Alcohol:* At site *Vehicles:* Up to 30 feet *Other:* Quiet hours 10 p.m.–7 a.m.; no motorboats on Buck Pond, only on Lake Kushaqua *Reservations:* 2-night stay required

MAP

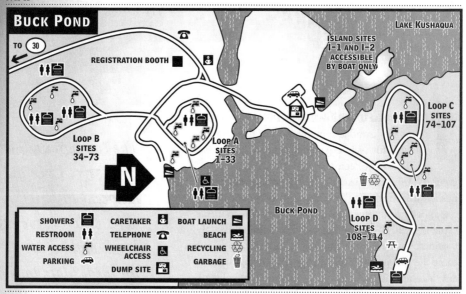

BUCK POND | LAKE KUSHAQUA

TO 30

REGISTRATION BOOTH

ISLAND SITES I-1 AND I-2 ACCESSIBLE BY BOAT ONLY

LOOP C SITES 74-107

LOOP B SITES 34-73

N

LOOP A SITES 1-33

BUCK POND

LOOP D SITES 108-114

SHOWERS		CARETAKER		BOAT LAUNCH	
RESTROOM		TELEPHONE		BEACH	
WATER ACCESS		WHEELCHAIR ACCESS		RECYCLING	
PARKING				GARBAGE	
		DUMP SITE			

GETTING THERE

From I-87 (Adirondack Northway), take Exit 30 to NY 73 North. Follow NY 73 North for 28 miles. In Lake Placid, take NY 86 West for 17 miles, passing through the village of Saranac Lake. In the village of Gabriels, turn right on NY 30. Follow NY 30 for 6 miles to the campground entrance on your left.

GPS COORDINATES

PARK ENTRANCE:
UTM Zone (WGS84)   18T
Easting   570183
Northing   4927313
Latitude   N 44°29'45"
Longitude   W 74°07'02"

and take in the impressive views of Big Haystack and Kate mountains.

Hiking is another attraction, with a popular short trail following the former rail bed. It's a little more than a mile to the outlet of Lake Kushaqua. For those looking to venture farther from camp, St. Regis Mountain in Paul Smiths and Debar Mountain at Meacham Lake are known for expansive vistas. Another option is the short but steep trail up Little Haystack. Be careful, though, because the trail is not very well marked.

One of the great things about the Adirondacks is its tradition of wilderness guides. For almost 200 years, these men and women have outfitted and led groups on trips in the woods, on the water, or both. Today, modern conveniences and technology make the wilderness more accessible to all, but that does not make it any less dangerous. Hiring an Adirondack guide is a great way to introduce yourself safely to a new area. When we visited Buck Pond, the caretaker informed us that he was licensed guide. It was pleasant to see a business card that summarizes one's offerings as "Fishing, Paddling, Photography, and Snowshoeing."

27
CRANBERRY LAKE
CAMPGROUND

THE RUGGED TERRAIN AND DENSE woodlands of the Adirondacks made most of the area inhospitable for Native Americans as well as for early settlers. The region served mostly as a battleground during colonization, and as farming settlements pushed westward after the American Revolution, the region lay mostly undiscovered. As the Industrial Age came into full swing, the region was exploited heavily for timber and minerals, but along with this exploitation came the region's first vacationers. Following their arrival, a growing acceptance of the inherent value of wilderness, along with a recognition of the devastation wrought by the demands of industry in the area, created a movement to preserve the remaining wilderness. Consequently, the Adirondack Forest Preserve was created with the intention to preserve the wild forests. The campgrounds at Cranberry Lake are adjacent to 150,000 acres of forest-preserve land, making it an ideal place to begin exploring the Adirondack wilderness.

The campground is laid out in two sections. The first, close to the entrance, is composed of the Upper Loop, Roadside Loop, Bear Mountain Loop, and Peninsula Loop. The second consists of Loops I through V. Campers will do best to skip sites along the Upper, Roadside, and Bear Mountain loops, because the majority are not as secluded, spacious, or scenic as sites along the other loops.

The Peninsula Loop sites (31 through 55) are well spaced, sit back from the road, and are surrounded by thick saplings, ferns, and other woodland vegetation. The southern part of the loop is adjacent to the lake, which becomes visible near site 40. A spur road with a tight turnaround heads left at this point, bringing you to sites 41 through 45. These sites hug the turnaround but have excellent views out to the lake. Complementing the views, the sites are larger than those encountered so far, but the canopy thins along the shore, so there is less brush between sites. Expansive views are also available from sites 46 through 48, but as the loop turns back toward the main road, they diminish.

> *The campgrounds at Cranberry Lake are adjacent to 150,000 acres of forest-preserve land, making it an ideal place to begin exploring the Adirondack wilderness.*

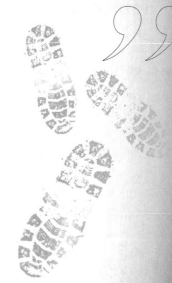

RATINGS

Beauty: ✿ ✿ ✿ ✿
Privacy: ✿ ✿ ✿
Quiet: ✿ ✿ ✿ ✿
Cleanliness: ✿ ✿ ✿
Security: ✿ ✿ ✿ ✿
Spaciousness: ✿ ✿ ✿

KEY INFORMATION

ADDRESS: Lone Pine Road
Cranberry Lake, NY
13064

OPERATED BY: New York State
Department of
Environmental
Conservation

INFORMATION: (315) 848-2315;
www.dec.state.ny.us/
website/do/camping

OPEN: Mid-May–
mid-October

SITES: 173 tent sites

EACH SITE HAS: Picnic table and
fire ring

ASSIGNMENT: Choose from
available sites or
reservations

REGISTRATION: 8 a.m.–9 p.m.

FACILITIES: Picnic areas,
amphitheater,
pavilion, potable
water, flush toilets,
swimming beach,
bathhouse, showers

PARKING: At site

FEE: $16/night most tent
sites; add $3/night
Friday, Saturday,
and holidays

ELEVATION: 1,547 feet

RESTRICTIONS: *Pets:* On leash
Fires: In fire rings
only
Alcohol: Allowed
Vehicles: RVs and
trailers limited to
specific sites
Other: Quiet hours
10 p.m.–7 a.m.;
6 people maximum/
site; maximum
14-night stay
Reservations: 2-night
stay required

However, the undergrowth thickens and the sites become even larger as you leave the loop.

A short drive south past the amphitheater and recycling and dump stations brings campers to Loops I through V. Although there is still a dense canopy of hardwoods, the brush between sites thins. Large boulders and a plethora of ferns dot the area, enhancing the wilderness setting. In general, the central sites are smaller and closer together than those on the perimeter along Loops I through III. Additionally, the first and last sites along these loops are near the main road, so they are also smaller and less desirable. Obviously, the best sites have views of the lake—along Loop I, these include sites 61 through 69. The sites on the perimeter here blend in with the rocky shore of the lake, providing picturesque campsites. Along Loop II, the sites with views of the lake begin at site 88 and end near site 98. Most sites along this loop are bigger than those described so far and will satisfy campers who desire more room. Loop III is elevated above its neighboring loops, and, consequently, partial views of the lake are present throughout. But the best lake views are from sites 117 through 124, because a tiny bay to the east partially surrounds these sites with water.

Loop IV essentially acts as the turnaround for the main road, so thru traffic is a minor concern here. The sites, however, are spacious, deep, and more spread out than in previous loops. Campers who prize space and solitude should look here, as the area is definitely less crowded with sites, and the feel of a deep woodland is pervasive. Loop V continues this remote wilderness setting but with less effect, as there are more sites and a small interior loop that brings central sites closer to each other and the main road.

Directly east of the campground is Bear Mountain, which can be reached by several trails. As you could guess, one trailhead is on the Bear Mountain Loop, and another is on Loop IV. From atop Bear Mountain, hikers can look out upon the Cranberry Lake and the vast forest preserves that await wilderness hikers. The Cranberry Lake Wild Forest, which surrounds the campground to the east and the lake to the west, has miles of hiking directly accessible from the campground. In addition, the Five Ponds Wilderness Area envelops the lake's southern shore and stretches miles to the west. Dozens of long trails can be reached from trailheads along CR 3 and adjoining roads, but some can also be

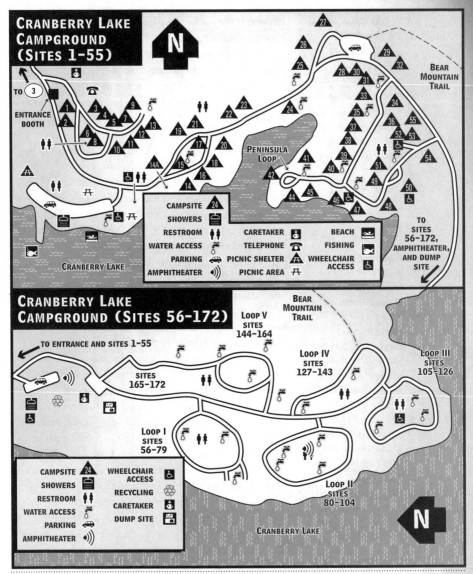

Cranberry Lake Campground (Sites 1–55)

N

TO **3**

ENTRANCE BOOTH

BEAR MOUNTAIN TRAIL

PENINSULA LOOP

CAMPSITE	24
SHOWERS	
RESTROOM		CARETAKER		BEACH	
WATER ACCESS		TELEPHONE		FISHING	
PARKING		PICNIC SHELTER		WHEELCHAIR ACCESS	
AMPHITHEATER	•)))	PICNIC AREA	

CRANBERRY LAKE

TO SITES 56–172, AMPHITHEATER, AND DUMP SITE

Cranberry Lake Campground (Sites 56–172)

BEAR MOUNTAIN TRAIL

TO ENTRANCE AND SITES 1–55

LOOP V SITES 144–164

LOOP IV SITES 127–143

LOOP III SITES 105–126

SITES 165–172

SITES 56–79

LOOP I SITES 56–79

LOOP II SITES 80–104

N

CRANBERRY LAKE

CAMPSITE	24	WHEELCHAIR ACCESS	
SHOWERS		RECYCLING	
RESTROOM		CARETAKER	
WATER ACCESS		DUMP SITE	
PARKING	
AMPHITHEATER	•)))

accessed by traversing Cranberry Lake by boat. A boat launch is located in the hamlet of Cranberry Lake, a short distance north of the campground, but campers along the shore could easily put in car-top boats directly from their sites.

GPS COORDINATES

UTM Zone (WGS84)	18T
Easting	513917
Northing	4893934
Latitude	N 44°11'55"
Longitude	W 74°49'33"

GETTING THERE

From I-81 North, take Exit 45, NY 3/Sackets Harbor/ Downtown. Turn right on NY 3 and drive a little more than 70 miles to Cranberry Lake Village. Turn right on Lone Pine Road and continue a little more than a mile to the park entrance.

28
EIGHTH LAKE

Views of the undeveloped and forested shores are exceptional— during the fall season they are emblazoned with color.

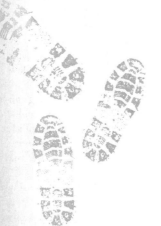

WHEN VISITORS COME to the Adirondacks, they are usually impressed with the sheer number of rugged hiking trails that criss-cross the wilderness. One of the other ways to explore this vast wilderness—which often escapes first-time visitors—is the numerous canoe routes. Interconnected rivers, streams, ponds, and lakes provide innumerable miles of adventure; and when connected by short portages, the distances canoes can travel are truly vast. Although the rivers and rapids in the Adirondacks should only be attempted by experienced boaters or with an outfitter, the placid lakes and ponds are within grasp of most novice boaters. Indeed, one of the more easily navigable canoe trips in the western Adirondacks is along the Fulton Chain of lakes. Roughly 20 miles long, part of this chain contains Seventh and Eighth lakes—the second and third largest as well as the least developed. Nestled between these two lakes is Eighth Lake Campground.

The campground is actually divided into three separate areas: one on the shores of Eighth Lake, one on the shores of Seventh Lake, and one (with a large number of sites) along the road between these areas. To access the sites along Eighth Lake's shore, drive past sites 1 though 9 (wooded and perfectly pleasant). Shaded by a mixture of pines and hardwoods, these sites have staggered drives and undergrowth for privacy. The next group of sites (11 through 20A) lies on an open lawn—although they back up to the woods, the woodland feel pervasive elsewhere in the campground is notably absent here. After passing these sites you have a choice: turn left and head to a group of sites within the shade of some very large pines (sites 46 through 54); or turn right along the lakeshore where the canopy becomes denser (sites 21 through 45). To the left, the tightly clustered group of sites is barely

RATINGS

Beauty: ✿ ✿ ✿ ✿
Privacy: ✿ ✿ ✿ ✿
Quiet: ✿ ✿ ✿ ✿
Cleanliness: ✿ ✿ ✿
Security: ✿ ✿ ✿
Spaciousness: ✿ ✿ ✿ ✿

separated from the day-use area by a log fence, making them very public and certainly not the choice for anyone seeking privacy.

Sites along the right fork and along the lakeshore side of the road are the real gems here and certainly the top choice of all the sites. Neighboring the boat launch for Eighth Lake, the first two sites (21 and 22) are more public than sites farther along the road. All the sites here are shaded by a mixture of hardwoods and softwoods, with lots of saplings and brush between. This, combined with ample space between sites, makes them ideal for campers seeking seclusion. Although sites across the road from the lake are nice woodland sites and offer glimpses of the lake, you can't beat the panoramic lake views seen from the shore. A thin belt of small hemlocks and other saplings encompasses the lakeside sites from the shore, but a short walk through this band of saplings takes campers directly to the lake. A narrow, sandy beach stretches along the shore to site 37, beyond which grasses and stones take over. Views of the undeveloped and forested shores are exceptional—during the fall season they are emblazoned with color.

The 1-mile-long road south to Seventh Lake (which is also the canoe portage between the two lakes) contains more than 40 woodland sites. In fact, the North Forest Canoe Trail, which connects the Fulton Chain of lakes to the northern tip of Maine via a 740-mile route through Vermont, Quebec, and New Hampshire, uses this road as a portage. Sites along this road blend into the forest, which transitions from dense pines along the western edge (found close to sites 55 through 68) to the more typical mixed-hardwood forest of the Adirondacks. All the sites in this area are large and well distributed along the road, and staggered drives help keep the area private despite a thin understory. Although most sites here are close to road, they become deeper as you approach the loop near Seventh Lake.

The sites maintain the deep woodland feel of the portage road until near site 110, where views of Seventh Lake add a new depth to the wilderness setting. From sites 110 through 119, all of the sites have good views

KEY INFORMATION

ADDRESS:	NY 28 Inlet, NY 13360
OPERATED BY:	New York State Department of Environmental Conservation
INFORMATION:	(315) 345-4120; www.dec.state.ny .us/website/do/ camping
OPEN:	Mid-May– Columbus Day
SITES:	126 tent sites
EACH SITE HAS:	Picnic table and fire ring
ASSIGNMENT:	Choose from available sites or reservations
REGISTRATION:	3 p.m.–9 p.m.
FACILITIES:	Picnic areas, potable water, flush toilets, boat launch, showers
PARKING:	At site
FEE:	$17/night most tent sites; add $3/night Friday, Saturday, and holidays
ELEVATION:	1,813 feet
RESTRICTIONS:	*Pets:* Dogs on leash with proof of currently valid rabies vaccination *Fires:* In fire rings only *Alcohol:* Allowed *Vehicles:* RVs and trailers allowed *Other:* Quiet hours 10 p.m.–7 a.m.; 6 people maximum/ site; maximum 14-night stay *Reservations:* 2-night stay required

MAP

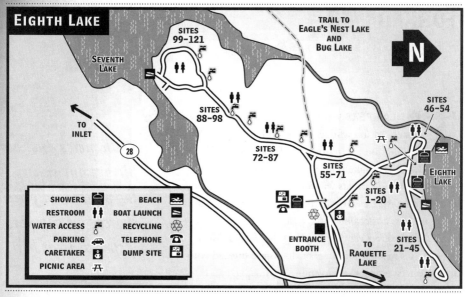

GETTING THERE

Use directions on page 88 through first sentence. Bear right onto NY 28 North and follow through Old Forge and Inlet. Continue along NY 28 North for another 6.7 miles. The campground entrance is on your left.

of the lake and a small, rugged island; at site 120, thick vegetation blocks the view. Generally the sites are a bit smaller here than elsewhere in the campground, but thicker brush enhances their privacy. Although all of the lakeside sites in this loop are close to the water and have magnificent views, of particular interest are sites 112 and 113, which are right on the water's edge. Note that the boat launch on this lake is close to sites 114A and 116, and don't forget to wave to the boaters on their way to Maine.

GPS COORDINATES

PARK ENTRANCE:

UTM Zone (WGS84) 18T
Easting   523752
Northing   4845908
Latitude   N 43°45'57"
Longitude   W 74°42'18"

29
FORKED LAKE

TENT CAMPERS WHO SEEK the solitude and beauty of the wilderness could hardly go wrong visiting the campground at Forked Lake. The rocky, 1,248-acre lake is an ideal boating and fishing spot, though motorboats will find navigating the shallow waters in North Bay treacherous. Indeed, scrape marks on numerous concealed rocks reveal that even shallow-draft canoes often get caught along the shores. Most approaches to sites' landings or docks are littered with these concealed rocks, warranting a slow pace and cautious eye. Since it is doubtful that boaters would wish to subject their propellers and deeper hulls to these numerous hazards and the trails between sites are very rugged, canoes or kayaks seem the more practical means of getting around the bay and campground in general. Fortunately, campers who don't own a boat can rent canoes right off a rack next to the boat launch.

The sites on Forked Lake are essentially boat-only sites, though the majority of them can be accessed along footpaths (3 through 34 and 63 through 76). A few sites (1, 2, 77 through 79) lie on an open lawn near the boat launch and are accessible to vehicles—but with so many other excellent sites, consider these only as a last resort. Encompassing the North Bay of Forked Lake, the lakeside sites afford phenomenal views. Going counterclockwise around the bay, campers pass several sites (3 through 7) that lie across the water from the boat launch. These sites are widely distributed among pines and short cedars, which seem to grow out of the rock-covered shores. For campers who don't have a boat or choose not to rent one, these will be the easiest sites to get to. Beyond site 7, the lake widens and you pass out of the visible range of the caretaker's cabin and any other vestiges of civilization. Along these rugged shores, the sites (8 through 15) become even more spread out as they continue west and then wrap

> *With views due west, picturesque sunsets over the water and forested shores give campers a special treat here.*

RATINGS

Beauty: ✿ ✿ ✿ ✿ ✿
Privacy: ✿ ✿ ✿ ✿ ✿
Quiet: ✿ ✿ ✿ ✿ ✿
Cleanliness: ✿ ✿ ✿ ✿ ✿
Security: ✿ ✿ ✿ ✿
Spaciousness: ✿ ✿ ✿ ✿

KEY INFORMATION

ADDRESS:	2 Forked Lake Road Long Lake, NY 12847
OPERATED BY:	New York State Office of Parks, Recreation and Historic Preservation
INFORMATION:	(518) 624-6646; www.dec.state.ny.us/ website/do/camping
OPEN:	Mid-May–Labor Day
SITES:	80 tent sites
EACH SITE HAS:	Fire ring and bear box
ASSIGNMENT:	Choose from available sites or reservations
REGISTRATION:	3 p.m.–9 p.m.
FACILITIES:	Pit toilets, boat launch
PARKING:	Near the boat launch
FEE:	$14/night most tent sites; add $3/night Friday, Saturday, and holidays
ELEVATION:	1,755 feet
RESTRICTIONS:	*Pets:* Dogs on leash with proof of currently valid rabies vaccination *Fires:* In fire rings only *Alcohol:* Allowed *Vehicles:* RVs and trailers limited to specific sites *Other:* Quiet hours 10 p.m.–7 a.m.; 6 people maximum/ site; maximum 14-night stay *Reservations:* 2-night stay required

around a large rocky corner, where the sites sit higher above the lake. As the lakeshore turns nearly due north, the remaining sites (16 through 34) along the footpath become a little closer together. The sites are surrounded by tall pines and cedars, scrub, and an occasional hardwood extending its branches over the mostly open sites. These sites feel completely secluded and there is plenty of room to set up. With views due west, picturesque sunsets over the water and forested shores give campers a special treat here.

The first boat-only site (35) is also on the eastern shore but is separated from the footpath sites by a marshy area and a small stream. This huge site is neighbored on its west by a larger stream, and the bay in front is covered by lily pads. Past the thick spread of lily pads, the boat-only sites mix in with dense evergreens and moss-covered boulders along the rock-covered shores. Widely spaced along the western shore, the sites (36 through 49) are spacious and secluded. Site 39 is particularly isolated—it's at the tip of the mainland between a lily-pad bay to the north and a boulder-strewn bay to the south. The sunrise over distant mountains illuminates these sites, so early risers enjoy a wonderful scene out of their tent door. Those who cannot decide between stunning sunrises or majestic sunsets could pick one of the island sites (50 through 52) and get both. Site 50 has its own private, forested, rocky island, whereas sites 51 and 52 share a slightly larger tree-covered island.

Past the islands and along a narrower strip of water, where the lake snakes west into Plumley Bay, are the last few boat-only sites (53 through 62). Dense pines shade these shores, and although the sites are not as spacious or spread out as some of the others, no sites here drop below a rating of "very desirable." Around the point and facing Plumley Bay are sites 60 through 62: if it is possible to feel more remote within this campground, these sites will do the trick.

A footpath serves the last remaining sites, which are along the southern shore toward the boat launch and past the two islands. Evergreens grow tall here, making these forested sites the shadiest in the campground. With 12 sites spread over three-quarters of a mile, it's

MAP

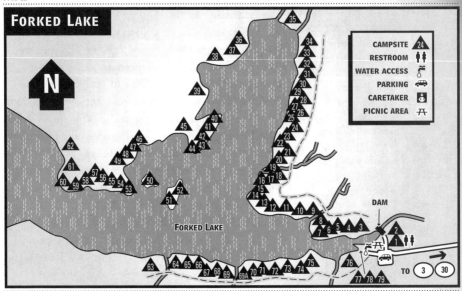

FORKED LAKE

CAMPSITE	🔺24
RESTROOM	👫
WATER ACCESS	🚰
PARKING	🚐
CARETAKER	🛖
PICNIC AREA	🏕

N

FORKED LAKE

DAM

TO 3 30

safe to assume you are guaranteed a private camping experience. Unique among these sites is site 75—large and grassy, with a sandy beach that faces west.

The only disclaimer for these wonderful sites is that they truly are primitive campsites, so visitors should be mindful of their impact on the area. Pit toilets are the only facilities available, and the bear boxes for food storage at each site clearly indicate the need for conscientious food and trash management. And because access to the sites is very limited, campground staff relies on strict compliance with carry-in, carry-out policy to ensure that the sites remain in their pristine state.

GETTING THERE

Use directions on page 88 through first sentence. Bear right onto NY 28 North. Pass Old Forge and Inlet; continue 23.7 miles. In Blue Mountain Lake, go straight on NY 28 North/NY 30 for 7.5 miles. Go left on CR 3. Go nearly 3 miles; at fork in road, go right on Forked Lake Road. Camp entrance is 1.8 miles ahead.

GPS COORDINATES

PARK ENTRANCE:

UTM Zone (WGS84)	18T
Easting	538043
Northing	4861454
Latitude	N 43°54'19"
Longitude	W 74°31'34"

If you have a tent and a boat, Indian Lake is the place to camp in the region.

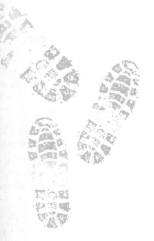

IN THE CENTRAL **ADIRONDACKS,** equidistant between the towns of Speculator and Indian Lake, are two distinct campgrounds. The first is Lewey Lake, an attractive group of sites located on or near the lake's 90 acres of water. The second is Indian Lake Islands, which is so close to Lewey that its entrance is located between Lewey's sites 35 and 37. The two offer very different camping experiences. Whereas Lewey has a beach, the standard amenities, and many waterfront sites among its 209, it can be congested and lacks the beauty of many other campgrounds in the mountains. Conversely, Indian Lake Islands has only 55 sites on its 4,000 acres, all with boat-only access, offering unparalleled privacy and amazing views. If you have a tent and a boat, Indian Lake is the place to camp in the region. Even if you don't have a boat, canoes and kayaks are available to rent from the Department of Environment Conservation (DEC) at the boat launch, and motorboats can be rented and delivered by marinas such as Dunn's Boat Service at Big Moose Lake. It would be hard to find an excuse not to visit.

Indian Lake is long and narrow, with more than 7 miles of water stretching between sites 1 and 51. At the southern end are three forks, the westernmost leading to Lewey Lake and the campground entrance. Development on the lake is concentrated on the northern end in the town of Sabael, where the rustic Timberlock family resort and a smattering of vacation homes line the water. Campers, however, will find the lake is rarely crowded, and the well-spaced sites are all solitary retreats unto themselves. To even reach the main section of sites, it is a 2.5-mile paddle from the registration booth.

Among the islands, five of the smaller ones house single sites and are perennially popular. These include

RATINGS

Beauty: ✿ ✿ ✿ ✿ ✿
Privacy: ✿ ✿ ✿ ✿ ✿
Quiet: ✿ ✿ ✿ ✿
Cleanliness: ✿ ✿ ✿ ✿
Security: ✿ ✿ ✿ ✿
Spaciousness: ✿ ✿ ✿ ✿ ✿

Kirpens Island (2), Crotched Pond Island (12), Moose Island (20), John Mac Bay (28), and a small nameless island off Long Island (32). Families and groups will often book neighboring sites at some of the multisite islands, including Doherty Island (7 and 8), Green Island (9 and 10), Camp Island (15 through 18) and Long Island (35 through 40), the largest of the bunch. Surprisingly, the most coveted site is not even on an island. Site 11, found near Watch Point, sits at the tip of a small peninsula, and promises campers their own beach and even a nearby waterfall.

Site 11 and the desirable island sites are often booked when they first become available—nine months in advance on ReserveAmerica (**www.reserveamerica .com**). But other lakeshore sites should not be overlooked. They are ideal for those of us who don't mark up calendars, and they tend to be more densely wooded, giving the impression of having the wilderness all to yourself. If you are looking for the quietest sites, consider 42 through 51, at the southernmost end of the lake. Many boats will pass by 52 through 55, but these four convenient sites are the closest to the registration booth and boat launch, a selling point for less-seasoned paddlers.

Canoes and kayaks are certainly popular, but motorboats can make distant points on the lake more accessible, and considering this is a carry-in, carry-out facility, they make ferrying supplies easier. There are no restrictions on the types of boats allowed, but there are also no docks at the sites. The lake is not marked: there are many submerged rocks. Losing a propeller is no way to start a camping trip. And be sure to arrive early. The steep launch is the only public one on the lake, so it gets plenty of day use and the parking lot can overflow.

Waterskiing is best enjoyed at the north end of the lake, but great fishing spots are everywhere. Trout, bass, and landlocked salmon attract many anglers. Some of the lakeshore is designated for picnicking, and both campers and day-use visitors take boats to trails that start right along the water's edge. On the eastern side of the lake are three 1-mile trails leading to Baldface Mountain, Crotched Pond, and Johnny Mack

KEY INFORMATION

ADDRESS:	General Delivery Sabael, NY 12864
OPERATED BY:	New York State Department of Environmental Conservation
INFORMATION:	(518) 648-5300; www.dec.state.ny .us/website/do/ camping
OPEN:	Mid-May–early September
SITES:	55
EACH SITE HAS:	Picnic table and fire ring
ASSIGNMENT:	Choose from available sites or reservations
REGISTRATION:	On arrival or by reservation (reserve minimum 2 nights)
FACILITIES:	Pit toilets
PARKING:	Central lot, near registration booth and boat launch
FEE:	$16/night
ELEVATION:	1,670 feet
RESTRICTIONS:	*Pets:* Dogs on leash with proof of currently valid rabies vaccination *Fires:* In fire rings only *Alcohol:* At site *Vehicles:* None permitted, all sites are boat access only *Other:* Quiet hours 10 p.m.–7 a.m.; carry out all trash *Reservations:* 2-night stay required

MAP

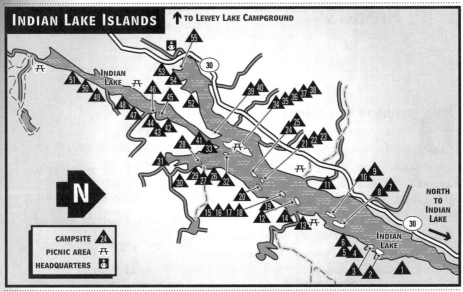

CAMPSITE 24
PICNIC AREA
HEADQUARTERS

GETTING THERE

From I-87 (Adirondack Northway), take Exit 23, Warrensburg. Follow US 9 North 4 miles to NY 28. Follow NY 28 West 33 miles. In Indian Lake Village, take NY 30 South 12 miles. Campground entrance is on the left.

GPS COORDINATES

PARK ENTRANCE:
UTM Zone (WGS84)   18T
Easting   549215
Northing   4833305
Latitude   N 43°39'04"
Longitude   W 74°23'23"

Pond. Just north of the campground entrance on Route 30 is a trail leading more than 4 miles to Snowy Mountain. Across the highway is the Watch Hill Trail, which climbs to great views of the lake on Watch Point.

Many campers on their way in or out of Indian Lake Islands take advantage of the showers, pay phone, and lifeguarded beach at Lewey Lake (no extra cost for those carrying their camping receipt). Others arriving too late to make their way to an Indian Lake site in the dark sometimes choose to use Lewey Lake as a stopover for the night. Just be warned that on summer weekends Lewey can fill to capacity, and you may have no choice but to find other accommodations.

Before the Indian Lake Islands campground officially opened in 1960, Indian Lake had long been home to informal campsites. Without supervision, heavy tree cutting, accumulation of trash, and forest fires left their scars on the shorelines. These days, under the watchful eye of the DEC, these problems are no longer common. Though it may seem inconvenient to haul your own trash, think of how much you appreciate pitching a tent at a clean, rustic site after a day of boating.

31
LAKE HARRIS

DRIVING TO LAKE HARRIS Campground on the curvy mountain road known as Route 28, look for signs depicting the silhouette of a man with glasses and a moustache. That's Theodore Roosevelt, all right. While camping on Mount Marcy on September 14, 1901, Teddy received word that President William McKinley had been shot and was not expected to recover. His party quickly hiked 10 miles down to Long Lake and Roosevelt continued west in a frantic nighttime stagecoach ride to the nearest train station. Arriving in North Creek, he discovered that McKinley had died and that he was in fact president. In commemoration of this legendary ride, Route 28 is now known as the Roosevelt-Marcy Trail. Roosevelt was of course a legendary outdoorsman and went on to become instrumental in the creation of the national park system. The Adirondacks didn't need his help, though. They were already preserved, thanks to a state law passed in 1885. The Adirondack Park continues to be larger than any national park in the continental United States.

Like many of the campgrounds in the region, Lake Harris offers waterfront sites, but in a much higher percentage than what is typically available. Almost two-thirds are along the water—57 out of 89— and all are well shaded by tall hardwoods. The first sites along the dirt road (1 through 5) are among the finest—large, private, and well spaced. More-congested spaces follow, but they are still adequately distributed, with sites 52 and 69 providing the most solitude. Sites 60, 76 through 79, 81, 83, and 90 are the least desirable, but the point is almost moot. Lake Harris is not among the most popular campgrounds in the Adirondacks, and except for holidays it is rarely busy. When reserving online, you currently cannot even choose specific sites. You will be informed as to how many

> *Lake Harris is one of the more convenient gateways to the southern end of the High Peaks Wilderness.*

RATINGS

Beauty: ☆ ☆ ☆ ☆
Privacy: ☆ ☆ ☆
Quiet: ☆ ☆ ☆ ☆
Cleanliness: ☆ ☆ ☆
Security: ☆ ☆
Spaciousness: ☆ ☆ ☆ ☆

KEY INFORMATION

ADDRESS:	Route 28 North Newcomb, NY 12852
OPERATED BY:	New York State Department of Environmental Conservation
INFORMATION:	(518) 582-2503; www.dec.state.ny.us/ website/do/camping
OPEN:	Mid-May–early September
SITES:	89
EACH SITE HAS:	Picnic table and fire ring
ASSIGNMENT:	Choose from available sites
REGISTRATION:	On arrival or by reservation (reserve minimum 2 nights)
FACILITIES:	Water, flush toilets, showers, pay phone
PARKING:	At site, maximum 2 vehicles
FEE:	$14/night
ELEVATION:	1,611 feet
RESTRICTIONS:	*Pets:* Dogs on leash with proof of currently valid rabies vaccination *Fires:* In fire rings only *Alcohol:* At site *Vehicles:* Up to 40 feet *Other:* Quiet hours 10 p.m.–7 a.m.; no swimming *Reservations:* 2-night stay required

sites are available in each loop, and you will be asked (sometimes in the form of a handwritten sign kindly posted at the registration booth) to choose your site when you arrive.

Fed by the northern part of the Hudson River, Lake Harris has 275 surface acres. While there is no swimming currently allowed at the campground, campers do certainly take advantage of the water. There is a small boat ramp just past the registration booth and larger public ramps elsewhere on the lake. Motorboats are allowed but only canoes and kayaks are available to rent. Smallmouth and largemouth bass, yellow perch, and northern pike will keep anglers casting their lines. Wildlife abounds in the surrounding woods, and although sightings of moose are extremely rare, bears are seen regularly. Please follow campground precautions concerning food storage and trash disposal.

Lake Harris is one of the more convenient gateways to the southern end of the High Peaks Wilderness, which has a major trailhead in Tahawus, about a 25-minute drive to the north. Some of the more celebrated hikes, such as Mount Marcy and Mount Algonquin, are closer to Lake Placid. Yet many folks will find it preferable to stay at Lake Harris and log a little time in the car in order to avoid the zoo that is Lake Placid in the summer. Closer to the campground, a 2-mile hike up Goodnow Mountain, capped by a fire tower, is a nice option for families who are ready for the 1,000-foot rise. The steepest part of the trail is in the beginning, and benches along the way provide convenient places to rest. Vanderwacker Mountain also has a fire tower, and at 5 miles round-trip is a little more challenging, but nothing more than a moderate day hike.

In addition to a monument commemorating Roosevelt's historic ride, there are a number of attractions in the vicinity of Lake Harris where you can learn more about the Adirondacks' 6 million acres. Newcomb houses one of the two Adirondack Park Interpretive Centers (the other is in Paul Smiths), where indoor exhibits are complemented by miles of surfaced nature trails. The Santanoni Preserve Historic

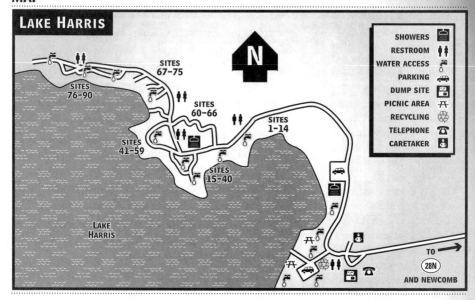

LAKE HARRIS

SITES 67–75
SITES 76–90
SITES 60–66
SITES 1–14
SITES 41–59
SITES 15–40

LAKE HARRIS

SHOWERS	
RESTROOM	
WATER ACCESS	
PARKING	
DUMP SITE	
PICNIC AREA	
RECYCLING	
TELEPHONE	
CARETAKER	

TO →
28N
AND NEWCOMB

Site can be reached by foot, bike, or car. A trail beginning at the edge of the campground leads 1.5 miles to the preserve and 6.5 miles to Santanoni's main lodge, or "great camp," which provides a fascinating perspective into the past, when the Adirondacks were being discovered as a playground for the rich who wanted the amenities of large homes but the feeling of true wilderness. During the summer, a number of the buildings are open to visitors, while the preserve itself is open year-round. Finally, 25 miles to the west in Blue Mountain Lake, you can visit the Adirondack Museum. This open-air museum includes 20 buildings, with exhibits depicting the rough-and-tumble history and culture of the mountains.

With the High Peaks close at hand and so many opportunities to learn about the natural and human history of the Adirondacks, Lake Harris is an ideal campground for both the curious and the adventurous. You may not stick around your tent for long, but when you do, you will appreciate the serene wilderness that attracted Roosevelt and so many others over the years.

GETTING THERE

From I-87 (Adirondack Northway), take Exit 23 to NY 28. Follow NY 28 northwest to North Creek. In North Creek, take NY 28 North to Newcomb. Campground entrance is on right.

GPS COORDINATES

PARK ENTRANCE:
UTM Zone (WGS84) 18T
Easting   570217
Northing   4869495
Latitude   N 43°58'31"
Longitude   W 74°07'28"

Lake George stretches through the southwestern Adirondacks like a wisp of smoke.

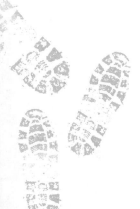

MANY PEOPLE'S CHILDHOOD MEMORIES of the Adirondacks revolve around the long and narrow Lake George. Its proximity to Albany, New York City, and even Boston (about 200 miles away) has made it an extremely popular summer getaway. Children's summer camps, rental cottages, lodges, and many budget motels line the lake's shores, and the water itself delights boaters of all stripes. 32 miles long and 3 miles wide at its widest point, Lake George stretches through the southwestern Adirondacks like a wisp of smoke. And islands, some acres-large and others little more than rocks sprouting a few trees, pop up across the water. You could camp along the shores at Roger's Rock or Hearthstone Point, but with almost 400 prime campsites to choose from on the lake's roughly 150 islands, why bother?

Lake George Islands is actually divided into the three campgrounds (or groups) with three separate headquarters. But it is hard to choose one group over another, and each site offers an equally memorable camping experience. With private docks and well-maintained pit toilets, this is primitive camping at its best.

On the southern end of the lake, not far from the town of Lake George, is the Long Island group, featuring 90 campsites. All sites are located on Long Island, which is large and shaped like a turkey leg. There are some small islands nearby for exploring and picnicking, including Diamond and Specker Heck, which have day-use areas—but your tent will have to stay put on Long Island. This does not mean you will feel cramped and overrun with neighbors. The campground staff has done a great job throughout the lake keeping all the islands well wooded and the sites well spaced. You will see other campers during your visit to Long Island, but this will not distract from the beauty of the surroundings.

RATINGS

Beauty: ✪ ✪ ✪ ✪ ✪
Privacy: ✪ ✪ ✪ ✪
Quiet: ✪ ✪ ✪ ✪
Cleanliness: ✪ ✪ ✪ ✪
Security: ✪ ✪ ✪ ✪ ✪
Spaciousness: ✪ ✪ ✪ ✪ ✪

Farther north, in The Narrows of the lake, is the Glen Island group. With its central location and 170 sites, it tends to be quite busy. Single-site islands (Bass, Gourd, Hermit, Little Gourd, Perch, Pine, Refuge, and Sunny) are unquestionably prime property. But the larger islands, such as Burnt with its 28 sites and Turkey with its 33, tend to be easier to book in advance. The group also features the lake's only cruiser sites. Located along the eastern shore at Red Rock Bay and on Log Bay Island, these 42 sites feature larger docks, designed for boats with sleeping quarters. Think of this as the RV section of the lake. Tent campers need not bother booking any of these—this area is mainly for people who want to sleep in the cabins of their boats.

The 85 sites of the Narrow Island Group are actually located north of The Narrows, which may be a little confusing. Just remember that this group (aka the Mother Bunch), stretches throughout the entire north half of the lake from just south of Huletts Landing almost the entire way to Ticonderoga. The islands are smaller in this neck of the water, and although single-site islands (Coopers, Horicon, Litburgess, Mallory, Phenita, and Steere) should not be passed up, only St. Sacrament, with 19 sites, could even be close to crowded.

Describing each individual site on Lake George would require an entire book. ReserveAmerica, which improved its Web site immeasurably in 2006, has done some of the work for us and provides distinct descriptions of each campsite, including details about water depth, foliage, and views. Pay careful attention to these options if you require a tent platform or have certain requirements for your boat. And a handful of sites are nonreservable—good for last-minute planners.

Before choosing a site, you should assess what your boat can handle. Although kayaks and canoes are common on Lake George, motorboats are the dominant form of transport. When the weather gets dicey, the wind often kicks up whitecaps on the lake, and paddlers may find themselves in danger. Campground staff told us tales of people with kayaks and canoes being stranded at their sites because of bad weather.

All three campground headquarters are located on islands (Glen, Long, and Narrow): you may have to

KEY INFORMATION

ADDRESS:	18 Boathouse Lane Bolton Landing, NY 12814
OPERATED BY:	New York State Department of Environmental Conservation
INFORMATION:	GI, (518) 644-9696; LI, (518) 656-9426; NI, (518) 499-1288; www.dec.state.ny.us
OPEN:	Mid-May–early September (LI), mid-September (NI), or early October (GI)
SITES:	GI, 212; LI, 90; NI, 85
EACH SITE HAS:	Picnic table, fire ring, dock, and toilet facility; 42 sites for large boats with sleeping quarters also have charcoal burners and pit toilets
ASSIGNMENT:	Choose from available sites or reservations
REGISTRATION:	On arrival or by reservation
FACILITIES:	Water, pit and flush toilets
PARKING:	At private marinas; fee usually charged
FEE:	$18/night
ELEVATION:	320 feet
RESTRICTIONS:	*Pets:* No dogs *Fires:* In fire rings only *Alcohol:* At site *Vehicles:* Boats only *Other:* Quiet hours 10 p.m.–7 a.m.; carry out all trash *Reservations:* GI and NI, 3-night stay required (LI, 1-night stay allowed)

MAP

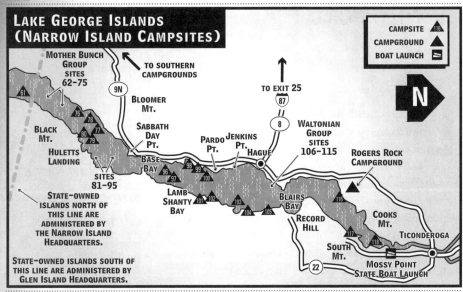

LAKE GEORGE ISLANDS (NARROW ISLAND CAMPSITES)

CAMPSITE
CAMPGROUND
BOAT LAUNCH

MOTHER BUNCH GROUP SITES 62-75

TO SOUTHERN CAMPGROUNDS

TO EXIT 25

61

9N

BLOOMER MT.

8

WALTONIAN GROUP SITES 106-115

76

78

BLACK MT.

80

77

79

SABBATH DAY PT.

PARDO PT.

JENKINS PT.

HAGUE

ROGERS ROCK CAMPGROUND

HULETTS LANDING

BASE BAY

96

38

99

100

SITES 81-95

97

STATE-OWNED ISLANDS NORTH OF THIS LINE ARE ADMINISTERED BY THE NARROW ISLAND HEADQUARTERS.

LAMB SHANTY BAY

101

102

103

104

105

116

BLAIRS BAY

RECORD HILL

COOKS MT.

TICONDEROGA

117

118

SOUTH MT.

22

MOSSY POINT STATE BOAT LAUNCH

STATE-OWNED ISLANDS SOUTH OF THIS LINE ARE ADMINISTERED BY GLEN ISLAND HEADQUARTERS.

N

GETTING THERE

Drive to Lake George from I-87 (Adirondack Northway) using Exits 21–25 and 28, then NY 9, NY 9N, NY 8, or NY 74. Contact a local marina for specific directions to chosen boat launch (see lower right).

travel a few miles over open water to check in, and then another few miles to get to your site. Be sure to leave yourself plenty of time—you don't want to rush, especially late in the evening or if you are not confident in your boating abilities. There are no official boat launches to access any of the campgrounds. The best option is to find a local marina and pay a small fee to park and launch. If you are renting a boat, this makes things quite convenient. But if you are bringing your own, it is a bit of an annoyance. Make sure to pick up a map and/or hydrographic chart at the marina, because the lake does hold many submerged rocks. For information on marinas, contact the campground offices or the Warren County Tourism Department, (518) 761-6366.

GPS COORDINATES

LONG ISLAND HEADQUARTERS:	GLEN ISLAND HEADQUARTERS:	NARROW ISLAND HEADQUARTERS:
UTM Zone (WGS84) 18	UTM Zone (WGS84) 18	UTM Zone (WGS84) 18
Easting 608871	Easting 612984	Easting 620418
Northing 4815507	Northing 4825414	Northing 4833617
Latitude N 43°29'04"	Latitude N 43°34'23"	Latitude N 43°38'45"
Longitude W 73°39'13"	Longitude W 73°36'03"	Longitude W 73°30'25"

33
LINCOLN POND

LINCOLN **P**OND **AND ITS SMALL** campground are located just east of the Adirondack Northway (Interstate 87). Surrounded by privately owned land, the pond and campground offer few trails for hikers (you will have to travel west into the Giant Mountain Wilderness to summit a few peaks). What they do offer, however, are some of the most beautiful campsites in the state.

A causeway separates Lincoln Pond into Upper and Lower Ponds, connecting the land at a narrow point. From here, some of the campsites are visible, while "camps," the Adirondack term for summer homes or cottages, can be seen across the water. The terminology dates back to the early 1800s, when Americans first discovered the joys of the Adirondacks, which were becoming an increasingly accessible wilderness. Even the grandest compounds are still called camps, but thankfully most of the camps on Lincoln Pond are just modest family homes. The famed "great camps," the grandest of these compounds, are farther to the west. So don't be confused if a local tells you he or she is "going to camp" for the weekend. They may have no intention of pitching a tent or firing up an RV.

A kayak, canoe, or small motorboat will undoubtedly enhance a visit to Lincoln Pond. Its gentle waters are great for an afternoon paddle or fishing for smallmouth bass, tiger muskie, and bullhead. There is no need to worry if you do not own a boat. The campground rents canoes and rowboats for a reasonable fee ($15 per day). You should worry about reservations, though. For although the main campground is full of fine waterfront sites, it is the interior sites that make it worth a visit.

With the exception of site I-10, each of the other nine interior sites borders the water. The closest of these to the main campground are I-1 through I-3,

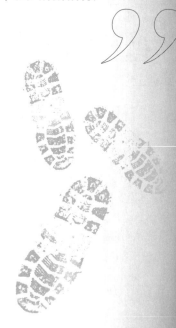

> *Campers can exit the major highway and be setting up tents within 30 minutes.*

RATINGS

Beauty: ✿ ✿ ✿
Privacy: ✿ ✿ ✿
Quiet: ✿ ✿ ✿
Cleanliness: ✿ ✿ ✿ ✿
Security: ✿ ✿ ✿ ✿
Spaciousness: ✿ ✿ ✿

accessible by car from Lincoln Pond Road. Of the first three, I-3 is the most private. Each site is also primitive, with a picnic table, fire ring, and pit toilets, but no running water. Campers have to return to the main area for water or a shower. This is a mild hassle and a short drive, but well worth it for the isolation. Three more of the interior sites (I-4 through I-6) are located on a small wooded island on Upper Pond, and boaters book these far in advance. Less than 2 miles down Lincoln Pond Road, turn right onto Kingdom Dam Road and drive for about 1 mile to reach sites I-7 through I-10. These are all excellent places to pitch a tent, but if we had to choose one site, it would be I-9. Perched on soft earth above the northern end of Lincoln Pond, it offers wonderful views, easy access to the water, and a spacious spot to hang a hammock, stow a boat, and enjoy a quiet day.

Back at Lincoln Pond's main camping area, you can take advantage of the day-use beach, picnic area, and car-top boat launch. Two nearby DEC campgrounds, Sharp Bridge and Crown Point (which share a brochure with Lincoln Pond because of their relatively small size), do not offer swimming, so some of their campers are likely to join locals at the beach here on hot days. The sand slopes down to the water and there are some very attractive spots to hunker down in a lawn chair and enjoy the surroundings.

The 25 sites in the main campground are rather open, with the waterfront sites being the least private (only a few birches and pines separate campers from their neighbors). But considering you can basically dip your feet in the water from these sites, try to reserve ahead (recommended for all sites on weekends and holidays) for 1, 2, 4, 6, 7, 9, 10, 12, 13, or 15. The last site along the water, 15, is spacious but very close to the causeway. Number 12 is on an embankment, so it is flat. The sites not directly on the water are also flat, but perched upon a slope, providing water views. The most private sites are 21 and 22. Site 23 is sunny and removed from the others, but is surrounded by an open field with an access road passing through, so it doesn't offer as much privacy as one might expect from the map.

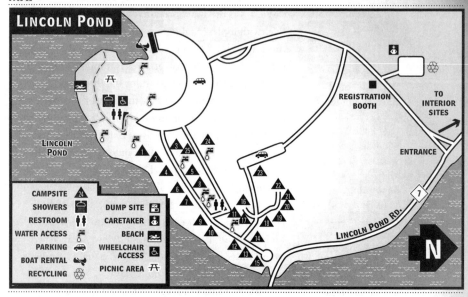

Nearby Elizabethtown is a good place to pick up supplies and is home to the Adirondack History Center, an excellent small museum. Here you'll find displays on recreation in the region and a number of restored vehicles, ranging from a brightly painted stagecoach to a hand-pump fire truck to a 1932 Olympics bobsled. One of its most popular attractions is the nearly 60-foot-high restored fire observation tower that you can climb for views of the town and the surrounding forest.

Bordered by I-87 to the west and Lake Champlain to the east, this section of the Adirondacks is more accessible than most. Campers can exit the interstate and be setting up tents within 30 minutes. And even with private "camps" on the shores of the lake, the sense of one's own space is still strong. Forest Preserve regulations limit development, and there are unlikely to be any major hotels constructed on the lake anytime soon. The privacy and accessibility of Lincoln Pond's interior sites make them even more desirable for tent campers. If you can plan ahead, it's worth the wait to get one of these well-planned spaces, whether for a couple's weekend getaway or a two-week family vacation.

GETTING THERE

From I-87 (Adirondack Northway), take Exit 31, Elizabethtown, and follow NY 9N west 4 miles. Turn left on CR 7 (Lincoln Pond Road) and go 6 miles to the campground entrance on the right.

GPS COORDINATES

PARK ENTRANCE:

UTM Zone (WGS84)   18T
Easting   613729
Northing   4888418
Latitude   N 44°08'24"
Longitude   W 73°34'41"

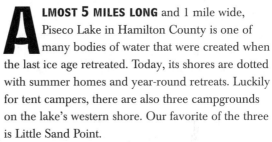

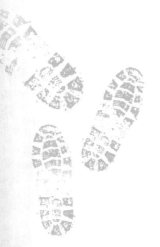

It is likely that campers will have the concrete boat ramp and sandy beach all to themselves.

ALMOST **5 MILES LONG** and 1 mile wide, Piseco Lake in Hamilton County is one of many bodies of water that were created when the last ice age retreated. Today, its shores are dotted with summer homes and year-round retreats. Luckily for tent campers, there are also three campgrounds on the lake's western shore. Our favorite of the three is Little Sand Point.

Poplar Point, near the northwestern corner of Piseco, is the smallest and oldest of the three, and features pit toilets and 24 sites along marshy water. It was built in 1927 and became so popular that the Department of Conservation quickly built Point Comfort, an area on the southwestern corner of the lake with composting toilets and 76 sites crowded together in what looks like a large picnic area. The aptly named Little Sand Point, built in 1953 and located between the other two, has the smallest beach and some relatively small sites, but it has the prettiest views, the most privacy, and the newest facilities (flush toilets, if that matters to you). We recommend you choose Little Sand for a stay on Piseco. All three campgrounds offer boat launches and beaches, but Little Sand is the farthest from town, and its facilities are rarely visited by day-trippers, so it is likely that campers will have the concrete boat ramp and sandy beach all to themselves.

Across from the entrance to the campground is the recycling center and dump station, wisely separated from the main area by County Route 8. The registration booth sits just past the gate, and a single road follows the shoreline past all 78 sites, with a circle at the far end to turn around. Slightly more than half of the spaces border the water, but trees block some of the views. These mixed hardwoods and conifers contribute a great deal of shade and a strong sense of privacy. And if the sites seem small at first in comparison to other campgrounds

RATINGS

Beauty: ✩ ✩ ✩
Privacy: ✩ ✩ ✩ ✩
Quiet: ✩ ✩ ✩ ✩ ✩
Cleanliness: ✩ ✩ ✩ ✩
Security: ✩ ✩
Spaciousness: ✩ ✩ ✩

in the Adirondacks, you will quickly find them to be more than adequate for a tent or two.

The first couple of sites are situated a little too close to the beach and boat ramp for comfort. Skip those. Most any of the other lakeside sites will do, and even though a hill gently slopes down the water, the sites themselves are flat. If you have your choice, try sites 50 through 65, the best for tents at Little Sand. Large rocks block the entrances to these sites, preventing cars from entering. Campers park along the road and walk the ten yards or so to pitch a tent. Vehicles are still easily accessible, but anyone camping in this section can be guaranteed a bit more privacy.

The nearby village of Piseco offers few supplies. Drive a little farther to Speculator, where the kitschy WELCOME TO SPECULATOR—ALL-SEASON VACATIONLAND sign greets you. It is one of area's larger villages, but considering that the population hovers around 350, that is not saying a heck of a lot. Still, there are spots for lunch and dinner, and a handful of inns and motels. It is a community that depends on outside visitors.

Closer to the campground, along County Route 8, a short trail affords excellent views of Piseco Lake. It meanders for about 0.8 miles up to Panther Mountain's 700-foot-high Echo Cliffs. The 5-mile T Lake Trail, climbing nearly 1,000 feet from Poplar Point Campground, might be a better choice for those looking for longer distances. And, if that's not enough for you, hop on a section of 133-mile Northville–Placid Trail at the northern tip of the lake. You'll be catching it at about the 30-mile point, so there is plenty more ground to cover.

Many campers (and others) take advantage of the lake and choose to fish for dinner or just for fun. Lake and brook trout, common and round whitefish, brown bullhead, chain pickerel, yellow perch, smallmouth bass, yellow perch, and pumpkinseed are all found in Piseco Lake. The lake itself can accommodate all sorts of boats. Motorboats, sailboats, canoes, and kayaks skim along the water on fine summer days. If campers get bored with the beach at Little Sand Point, they can enjoy the sometimes-quieter Poplar Point Beach or the busier Point Comfort Beach. But always check in advance

KEY INFORMATION

ADDRESS:	Old Piseco Road Piseco, NY 12139
OPERATED BY:	New York State Department of Environmental Conservation
INFORMATION:	(518) 548-7585; www.dec.state.ny .us/website/do/ camping
OPEN:	Mid-May–early September
SITES:	78
EACH SITE HAS:	Picnic table and fire ring
ASSIGNMENT:	Choose from available sites or reservations
REGISTRATION:	On arrival or by reservation (reserve minimum 2 nights)
FACILITIES:	Water, flush toilets, showers, pay phone
PARKING:	At site, maximum 2 vehicles
FEE:	$16/night
ELEVATION:	1,668 feet
RESTRICTIONS:	*Pets:* Dogs on leash with proof of currently valid rabies vaccination *Fires:* In fire rings only *Alcohol:* At site *Vehicles:* Up to 30 feet *Other:* Quiet hours 10 p.m.–7 a.m. *Reservations:* 2-night stay required

MAP

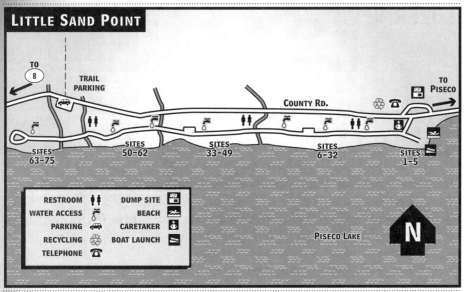

LITTLE SAND POINT

TO 8

TRAIL PARKING

COUNTY RD.

TO PISECO

SITES 63–75

SITES 50–62

SITES 33–49

SITES 6–32

SITES 1–5

RESTROOM	DUMP SITE
WATER ACCESS	BEACH
PARKING	CARETAKER
RECYCLING	BOAT LAUNCH
TELEPHONE	

PISECO LAKE

N

GETTING THERE

From I-90 (New York State Thruway), take Exit 27, Amsterdam, to NY 30 North. Follow NY 30 North for 50 miles. In Speculator, turn left on NY 8 West. After 11 miles, turn right on Old Piseco Road, and follow it for 5 miles. Campground entrance is on the left.

GPS COORDINATES

PARK ENTRANCE:

UTM Zone (WGS84)   18T
Easting   536303
Northing   4807290
Latitude   N 43°25'03"
Longitude   W 74°33'06"

to see if any lifeguards are on duty—they can be hard to come by in this neck of the woods.

Private homes share the western edge of the lake with the campground. You may spy summer visitors looking out over the blue water and green forests from their comfortable, weathered Adirondack chairs. It is easy to see why this characteristic type of outdoor furniture, with its sloping back and wide armrests, is named after the region: an Adirondack chair, like the mountains themselves, evokes a slow pace and simple, natural pleasures. Back at Sandy Point, you may have to make due with a well-worn picnic-table bench. It's a small sacrifice for a quiet night in this pleasant little getaway on the water.

STRADDLING THE "BLUE LINE" marking the border of the Adirondack Park, the town of Lake Luzerne is known as the "Gateway to the Adirondacks," and Luzerne campground is just inside this boundary. Like much of the area, the surrounding forest was once owned by a lumber company and heavily logged in the 1940s and 1950s. When the state purchased the land in the 1960s, horse trails were already established on the property. Now the trees are thick again, and this pleasant campground has the unique features of horse camping and two separate swimming areas—one reserved for campers only.

After entering Luzerne, turn left and pass the boat launch to reach the campsites. The first section (sites 1 through 14) is set in dense, shady forest with beds of pine needles that seem to be inviting you to unpack your tent. Removed from the other loops, this section undoubtedly ensures the most quiet. Sites 7 through 11, down a short hill on a small secluded spur, are the ones to choose here. Skip sites 4 and 12 through 15, which are a little too close to the road. Beyond the first section, the camp road curves, crossing a stream and the "Field of Dreams," a grassy clearing perfect for a lazy picnic. The next section of sites (15 through 37) is larger and also isolated, but draws bigger crowds. Ferns are thick in this section, and site 22, carved a little deeper in the forest, was our favorite here.

Another short drive down the road is the next section, by far the largest, with more than half the sites in the entire campground. Sites 38 through 123 are arranged in a group of intersecting loops, and many centrally located spaces have their own entrances but neighbors on the other three sides. On the campground map, sites 81, 82, 113, 114, 116, and 118 appear to be close to the water's edge and the beach, so they tend to book up quickly. But they are atop a steep hill. Don't

> *Two corrals, a barn, and miles of horse trails round out the benefits for equestrians.*

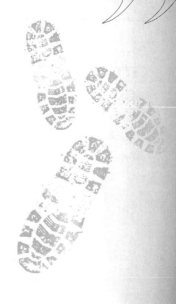

RATINGS

Beauty: ✩ ✩ ✩
Privacy: ✩ ✩ ✩
Quiet: ✩ ✩ ✩ ✩
Cleanliness: ✩ ✩ ✩
Security: ✩ ✩ ✩
Spaciousness: ✩ ✩ ✩

ADDRESS: 892 Lake Avenue
(NY 9N)
Lake Luzerne, NY
12846

OPERATED BY: New York State
Department of
Environmental
Conservation

INFORMATION: (518) 696-2031;
www.dec.state.ny.us/
website/do/camping

OPEN: Mid-May–early
September

SITES: 174

EACH SITE HAS: Picnic table and
fire ring

ASSIGNMENT: Choose from
available sites or
reservations

REGISTRATION: On arrival or by
reservation (reserve
minimum 2 nights)

FACILITIES: Water, flush
toilets, hot showers,
pay phone

PARKING: At site, maximum
2 vehicles

FEE: $18/night

ELEVATION: 620 feet

RESTRICTIONS: *Pets:* Dogs on leash
with proof of
currently valid
rabies vaccination;
horses require proof
of currently valid
Coggins test
Fires: In fire rings
only
Alcohol: At site
Vehicles: Up to 30 feet
in main section,
up to 40 feet in horse
section
Other: Quiet hours
10 p.m.–7 a.m.
Reservations: 2-night
stay required

expect to fall asleep to the sound of lapping water here. Number 94 is one of the most private spots; 119, 120, and 120A are set off on a spur near a ravine.

From the small parking lot near site number 113, it's just a 50-yard walk down to the camper's beach. This small patch of sand lies across the lake from the day-use bathing area. Both have lifeguards on duty during summer days. The camper's beach is the smaller of the two, but is quieter and has its own rowboats and canoes for rent. It is nice to see that your camping pass can get you more than just a patch of dirt and a fire pit. Even if you're not a sun worshipper, the beach is still a great place to take in the lovely views of the wooded slopes surrounding the water.

Leaving the main group of sites, you pass the campground's shower building. Comfort stations and water spigots are well spaced throughout the campground, but this is the only place for a shower, and thankfully it features a small parking lot. Turn right after the showers and on to the main road, and 124 through 150 are the next group of sites. Though these sites are nicely removed from the largest section, power lines crisscross overhead and seem incongruous to the surroundings. The sites would be quite pleasant if not for the constant reminder of civilization.

The final section is made up of the equestrian sites (H1 through H22). Although this area is essentially an open field surrounded by pines, campers with horses will appreciate not having to book extra sites. Two corrals, a barn, and miles of horse trails round out the benefits for equestrians. There are only 5 miles of equine trails within the surrounding public land, but more than 60 miles are accessible on adjacent private property—detailed on a posted map. On holiday weekends, you must have a horse to stay in this area.

The lake itself is known as Fourth Lake, a testament to the sheer number of lakes in the Adirondacks—they ran out of names and had to settle for numbers! Second and Third Lakes are to the south and Lake Luzerne is actually a separate and much larger body of water found in town. Fourth Lake is only partially bordered by the campground, but is still a quiet bit of water with no motorboats allowed. The day-use area

MAP

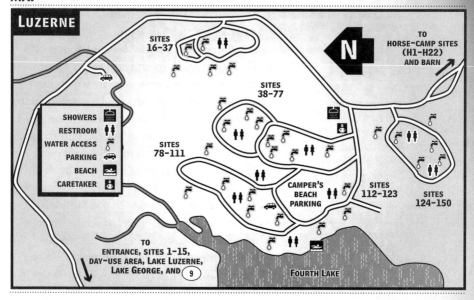

LUZERNE

SITES 16–37

TO HORSE-CAMP SITES (H1–H22) AND BARN

SITES 38–77

SHOWERS
RESTROOM
WATER ACCESS
PARKING
BEACH
CARETAKER

SITES 78–111

CAMPER'S BEACH PARKING

SITES 112–123

SITES 124–150

TO ENTRANCE, SITES 1–15, DAY-USE AREA, LAKE LUZERNE, LAKE GEORGE, AND 9

FOURTH LAKE

is popular for swimming, picnicking, and fishing. Canoes and rowboats are also available for rent at the beach. The park staff runs a nature recreation program—check the posted *Wilderness Times,* a summary of daily events written by the camp staff in the summer.

Even if you don't own a horse, you can still have a cowboy experience nearby. Just follow the Dude Ranch Trail signs north on 9N, and in minutes you'll be at the Painted Pony Rodeo. Barbecue dinners and rodeo shows rope in everyone from cowboys to greenhorns. For a shopping and dining blitz, continue on to Lake George and its honky-tonk attractions. There are campgrounds on the shores of Lake George, but they are even larger than Luzerne's, and tent campers should avoid them in summer (the Lake George Islands campgrounds, page 113, are another story). Luzerne is much quieter and almost as close to the action. If you avoid the largest section of sites, it's hard even to believe that you are camping in such a large campground. The facilities are well worn but clean, a testament to the many people who have enjoyed the campground over the years.

GETTING THERE

From I-87 (Adirondack Northway), take Exit 21 to NY 9 South. Follow NY 9 South 7 miles to the campground entrance on the left.

GPS COORDINATES

PARK ENTRANCE:

UTM Zone (WGS84)   18T
Easting   594422
Northing   4791875
Latitude   N 43°16'26"
Longitude   W 73°50'11"

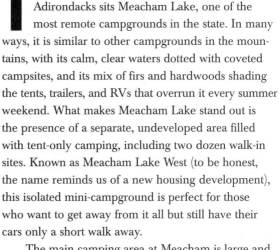

> *What makes Meacham Lake stand out is the presence of a separate, undeveloped area filled with tent-only camping, including two dozen walk-in sites.*

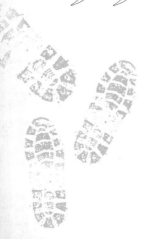

IN THE FAR NORTHWEST CORNER of the Adirondacks sits Meacham Lake, one of the most remote campgrounds in the state. In many ways, it is similar to other campgrounds in the mountains, with its calm, clear waters dotted with coveted campsites, and its mix of firs and hardwoods shading the tents, trailers, and RVs that overrun it every summer weekend. What makes Meacham Lake stand out is the presence of a separate, undeveloped area filled with tent-only camping, including two dozen walk-in sites. Known as Meacham Lake West (to be honest, the name reminds us of a new housing development), this isolated mini-campground is perfect for those who want to get away from it all but still have their cars only a short walk away.

The main camping area at Meacham is large and fairly standard, but we do not want to downplay its appeal. It includes a day-use area with a picnic shelter, sandy beach, playground, and canoes and rowboats for rent. Day-use visitors are scarce, as the closest major towns are Malone and Saranac Lakes (20 miles to the north and south, respectively), and campers rarely have to contend with crowds. One of the unique features of the campground is the large amphitheater found east of the beach, on the southern side of the shower-house parking lot. With seating for up to 100 people, it serves as a venue for educational and recreational activities (including movies and even the occasional karaoke session). For daily events in the summer, look for the posted *Wilderness Times* newsletter or talk to the camp staff.

If privacy is the most important aspect of a campsite for you, seek out sites 25 through 33, 72, or 73, which are spacious and set deeper into the woods than most. Avoid sites 1 through 5, 42 through 44, 53 through 55, and 84 through 91. They are crowded, and

RATINGS

Beauty: ✩ ✩ ✩ ✩
Privacy: ✩ ✩ ✩ ✩
Quiet: ✩ ✩ ✩ ✩
Cleanliness: ✩ ✩ ✩
Security: ✩ ✩ ✩ ✩
Spaciousness: ✩ ✩ ✩ ✩

not as shady as one might like. The waterfront sites (153 through 174) are certainly the most popular, and visitors will appreciate that there is no private development on the lake to spoil the views. Especially for waterfront sites, reservations on weekends and holidays are essential, but walk-in campers should not have problems during the week if they are happy with a standard site.

Surprisingly, according to camp staff, Meacham Lake West is the last area to fill up by advance request. Removed from the main campground and day-use area, it is about a mile past the boat ramp via a paved road with the occasional pothole. The road turns to dirt, and you have to park your car and hoof it to access some of the sites. If that's not enough to keep the trailers away, the fact that only one collection of pit toilets services the 50 sites will do the trick (more-convenient, but primitive, outhouses are scattered throughout the area).

Sites 175 through 199 are all primitive walk-in sites, but the walk to each varies from about 30 to 300 yards. All sites are either on the water or open to excellent views—each has its own pit toilet and tent platform. The facilities may be a little old, and the lakeshore sites are not completely private (other sites can often be seen through the trees), but they are a vast improvement over most accommodations a tent camper is likely to find. For those who would like to take advantage of the remoteness of Meacham Lake West, but would prefer the proximity of a few more amenities, sites 201 through 223 are spread out along a separate road and are closest to the toilets and a series of water spigots. Sites 179 through 181 sit atop a grassy hill and would be perfect for group camping.

A firewood and ice truck peddles the basics to campers once a day (more frequently in the summer). For other supplies, the closest store is a 6-mile drive north out of the campground along Route 30. But a little time on the road is not such a bad thing around here. New York's Route 30, a scenic byway known as The Adirondack Trail, is one of the nicest stretches of road in the state. Follow it almost 10 miles south to the village of Paul Smiths, home to Paul Smith's College,

KEY INFORMATION

ADDRESS:	P.O. Box 53 Paul Smiths, NY 12970
OPERATED BY:	New York State Department of Environmental Conservation
INFORMATION:	(518) 483-5116; www.dec.state.ny.us/website/do/camping
OPEN:	Mid-May–early October
SITES:	224 (48 primitive, including 24 walk-in)
EACH SITE HAS:	Picnic table and fire ring (walk-in sites also have tent platforms)
ASSIGNMENT:	Choose from available sites or reservations
REGISTRATION:	On arrival or by reservation
FACILITIES:	Water (potable water not available at walk-in sites), pit and flush toilets, showers, pay phone
PARKING:	At site or designated areas for walk-ins, maximum 2 vehicles
FEE:	$16/night
ELEVATION:	1,573 feet
RESTRICTIONS:	*Pets:* Dogs on leash with proof of currently valid rabies vaccination *Fires:* In fire rings only *Alcohol:* At site *Vehicles:* Up to 40 feet *Other:* Quiet hours 10 p.m.–7 a.m. *Reservations:* 1-night stay allowed

MAP

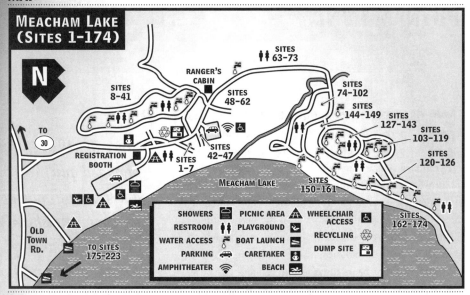

MEACHAM LAKE
(SITES 1-174)

N

TO
30

SITES
8-41

RANGER'S
CABIN

SITES
48-62

SITES
63-73

SITES
74-102

SITES
144-149

SITES
127-143

SITES
103-119

SITES
120-126

REGISTRATION
BOOTH

SITES
42-47

SITES
1-7

MEACHAM LAKE

SITES
150-161

SITES
162-174

OLD
TOWN
RD.

TO SITES
175-223

SHOWERS	PICNIC AREA	WHEELCHAIR ACCESS	
RESTROOM	PLAYGROUND		
WATER ACCESS	BOAT LAUNCH	RECYCLING	
PARKING	CARETAKER	DUMP SITE	
AMPHITHEATER	BEACH		

GETTING THERE

From I-87 (Adirondack Northway), take Exit 30 to NY 73 North. Follow NY 73 North for 28 miles. In Lake Placid, take NY 86 West for 22 miles, passing through the village of Saranac Lake. In Paul Smiths, turn right on NY 30 North. Follow NY 30 North for 9.5 miles. Campground entrance is on right.

GPS COORDINATES

PARK ENTRANCE:
UTM Zone (WGS84)   18T
Easting   556251
Northing   4937223
Latitude   N 44°35'10"
Longitude   W 74°17'29"

known for its programs in forestry, ecology, and hospitality. The village is also home to one of the two Adirondack Park Visitor Interpretive Centers (the other is in Newcomb), a great place to learn about the region through wildlife exhibits, scheduled events, and miles of surfaced trails designed for those not quite ready for backcountry hiking.

From Paul Smiths, hikers can strap on their boots and try to summit St. Regis Mountain, a 2,874-foot peak that overlooks the St. Regis Canoe Area. Those who would rather not drive to a trailhead can set off from the campground and climb Debar Mountain, a 7.4-mile round trip that will take you up to 3,200 feet, the best vantage point in the Debar Mountain Wild Forest.

While it may not be evident now, the campground was built on the site of a well-known regional hotel, which offered rooms to vacationers until 1921. The accommodations available at Meacham Lake these days are admittedly a bit more rustic, but the inviting sounds of nature and true feeling of wilderness should keep visitors coming back.

37
PUTNAM POND

FORT **TICONDEROGA,** **BUILT BY** the French (and formerly called Fort Carillon) in the 1750s, once was one of the most strategically important military sites in the New World. Located at the point where Lake Champlain meets Lake George, it was known as the "key to the continent" and changed hands for the next 20 years between the French, the British, and the Americans. In 1820, it was privately purchased, and preservation of the site began. The fort, and the town that bears it name, still remain—but now the region, with its shimmering bodies of water, is more notable as a summer getaway, and the number of nearby campgrounds speaks to that fact. Paradox Lake, Crown Point, and Rogers Rock all provide camping within minutes of Ticonderoga. But Putnam Pond, just 6 miles down the road, features the finest accommodations for the tent camper.

Putnam Pond, known locally as "Putts Pond," was originally named after General Israel Putnam, who gained notoriety as a captain who fought in the region during the French and Indian War and later commanded forces at Bunker Hill. Since the campground's construction in the early 1960s, it has provided quiet camping and tranquil waters for boaters wishing to escape the wakes of Lake George and Lake Champlain. Unlike many campgrounds in the Adirondacks, it does not offer waterfront sites in its main campground. However, it does have a handful of boat-in and walk-in sites along its shores, and campers snatch these up quickly.

Putnam Creek, which flows from a dam on the east side of the pond and eventually runs into Lake Champlain, welcomes visitors as they drive over a bridge just past the entrance. The first sites, 1 through 16, are perfectly adequate but are a bit too close to the road for our tastes. Sites 17 through 34, on the north

> *Since the 1960s, it has provided quiet camping and tranquil waters for boaters wishing to escape the wakes of Lake George and Lake Champlain.*

RATINGS

Beauty: ✰ ✰ ✰ ✰
Privacy: ✰ ✰ ✰ ✰ ✰
Quiet: ✰ ✰ ✰
Cleanliness: ✰ ✰ ✰ ✰
Security: ✰ ✰ ✰ ✰
Spaciousness: ✰ ✰ ✰

ADDRESS: 763 Putts Pond Road Ticonderoga, NY 12883

OPERATED BY: New York State Department of Environmental Conservation

INFORMATION: (518) 585-7280; www.dec.state.ny.us/ website/do/camping

OPEN: Mid-May–early September

SITES: 72 (9 interior sites only accessible by boat)

EACH SITE HAS: Picnic table and fire ring

ASSIGNMENT: Choose from available sites or reservations

REGISTRATION: On arrival or by reservation

FACILITIES: Water (potable water not available at interior sites), pit and flush toilets, showers, pay phone

PARKING: At site, maximum 2 vehicles or central lot for interior sites

FEE: $14/night

ELEVATION: 1,276 feet

RESTRICTIONS: *Pets:* Dogs on leash with proof of currently valid rabies vaccination
Fires: In fire rings only
Alcohol: At site
Vehicles: Up to 30 feet
Other: Quiet hours 10 p.m.–7 a.m.
Reservations: 1-night stay allowed

end of the campground, were what sold us on Putnam. We particularly liked site 28, which is shaded by large trees and set back along a slope, far from the road. Views of the pond are not as common as one might hope, but that enhances the feeling that you are in thick woods. For a glimpse of the water, choose sites 46 or 47. Groups and large RVs are often directed to a grassy circle of sites (58 through 61) on the south side of the park, well removed from everyone else. And three "management" sites are maintained and often used for overflow. During the week, walk-ups should not have trouble finding vacancies, but weekends and holidays fill up quickly.

When we asked a staff member which sites are the most popular, she showed us her reservation sheet. The sites most frequently marked as booked happened to be the least accessible of the bunch, at least for the unfortunate folks without a boat or a sturdy pair of boots. The campground manages nine interior pond sites, including one on a small island (I-5). It is possible but difficult to hike in to sites I-8 and I-9 on the pond's north shore, but the rest require something to float you and your stuff over. This is not Lake George; the waters are not exactly teeming with cabin cruisers. A canoe or kayak should do the trick. Remember, this is primitive camping, without a potable water source—but picnic tables, fire rings, and pit toilets are provided. With the isolation and the splendid view of Putnam, it's doubtful you'll miss flush toilets or hot showers during your stay.

Even if you have not reserved an interior site, a boat is certainly worth bringing. There are no restrictions on horsepower, but the pond is ideally suited for small motors and self-propelled crafts. Anglers, who cast for smallmouth bass and tiger muskies, will be pleased, while water-skiers will likely not be. The many ponds in the adjacent Pharaoh Mountain Wilderness offer long stretches of water for canoes, but those who wish to paddle in the remote woods should be prepared to portage at least half a mile to reach their destination.

Landlubbers need not worry. There are plenty of things to do on dry land. Trails to Rock Pond and

MAP

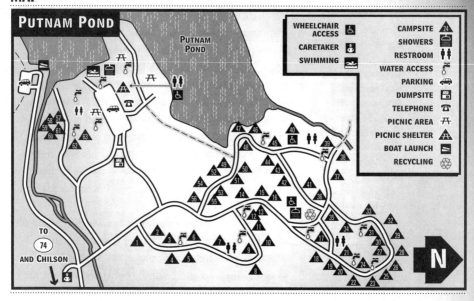

PUTNAM POND

PUTNAM POND

WHEELCHAIR ACCESS

CARETAKER

SWIMMING

CAMPSITE

SHOWERS

RESTROOM

WATER ACCESS

PARKING

DUMPSITE

TELEPHONE

PICNIC AREA

PICNIC SHELTER

BOAT LAUNCH

RECYCLING

TO **74** AND CHILSON

N

Treadway Mountain are easily accessible from a parking lot near the campground's boat launch. Many hikers set out on the Long Swing Trail for a day trip to the wonderfully named Grizzle Ocean, or soldier on for a multiday backpack to Pharaoh Lake, Pharaoh Mountain, and beyond. Lean-tos are distributed along the trails, but these are so often occupied that the campground serves as overflow for unlucky souls who cannot find a shelter in the backcountry.

Back in Ticonderoga, history buffs can learn about the area's role in the Revolution and in the French and Indian War. If Israel Putnam is to be believed, it was not far from here that he was once captured, tied to a tree and subjected to a game of William Tell by an overzealous Native American using a tomahawk instead of a bow and arrow. The only games that modern visitors need to fear are the ubiquitous mini-golf courses in nearby Lake George, the largest town in the Adirondacks. If you are like us, you'll prefer to stay close to Putnam Pond and enjoy the surrounding wilderness.

GETTING THERE

From I-87 (Adirondack Northway), take Exit 28. Take NY 74 East for 9 miles. Turn right on CR 39 (Putts Pond Road). Follow CR 39 for 4 miles to the campground entrance, straight ahead.

GPS COORDINATES

PARK ENTRANCE:

UTM Zone (WGS84)   18T

Easting   615180

Northing   4855130

Latitude   N 43°50'25"

Longitude   W 73°34'02"

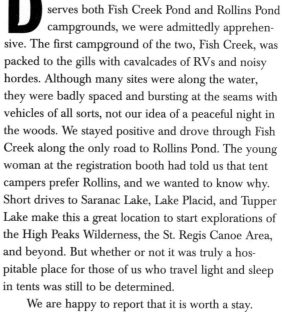

> *Rollins Pond, although busy in the summer, is hardly the zoo (or shall we say aquarium) that is Fish Creek Pond.*

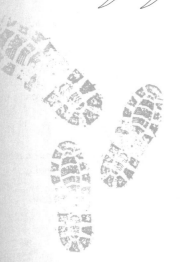

DRIVING THROUGH THE ENTRANCE booth that serves both Fish Creek Pond and Rollins Pond campgrounds, we were admittedly apprehensive. The first campground of the two, Fish Creek, was packed to the gills with cavalcades of RVs and noisy hordes. Although many sites were along the water, they were badly spaced and bursting at the seams with vehicles of all sorts, not our idea of a peaceful night in the woods. We stayed positive and drove through Fish Creek along the only road to Rollins Pond. The young woman at the registration booth had told us that tent campers prefer Rollins, and we wanted to know why. Short drives to Saranac Lake, Lake Placid, and Tupper Lake make this a great location to start explorations of the High Peaks Wilderness, the St. Regis Canoe Area, and beyond. But whether or not it was truly a hospitable place for those of us who travel light and sleep in tents was still to be determined.

We are happy to report that it is worth a stay. Rollins Pond, while busy in the summer, is hardly the zoo (or shall we say aquarium) that is Fish Creek Pond. This may be because there are no day-use facilities and no beach (Fish Creek serves that purpose). It may also be because there are fewer waterfront sites at Rollins and a restriction on boat-motor size. Or it may be the longer drive—a 10-mile-per-hour slog past almost 200 of Fish Creek's sites—that turns some away. Whatever the reason, it is all a blessing.

While you must pass through the entrance of Fish Creek to get to Rollins Pond, you will have to check in at another registration booth once you reach the campground. Just past the booth, on the southern side of the pond, are the well-spaced waterfront sites, A1 through A31, some of the nicest in the campground (there is also A32, but it is an interior site and worth a pass). In general, the best sites are on the southern side of the

RATINGS

Beauty: ✿ ✿ ✿
Privacy: ✿ ✿ ✿
Quiet: ✿ ✿
Cleanliness: ✿ ✿ ✿
Security: ✿ ✿ ✿ ✿
Spaciousness: ✿ ✿ ✿

pond, and it would also be hard to go wrong choosing from sites 1 through 52, many of which are located directly along the pond's shores (sites 24, 26, 29, 31, 33, 39, 44, 46, and 49 are all interior sites, but often open onto views of the water). All sites in the campground are shaded by a mix of firs and hardwoods.

The central section of the campground, particularly sites 53 through 107, is more crowded, and most sites here are located along the edge of a slope that leads down to the water. If you can, choose a site in another section. Farther north along the water, sites in the 140s open onto a small beach. With the exception of 102, 103, and 252 through 257, which are not as private as one might wish, almost any site found farther north along the pond is a good choice. When placing a reservation on ReserveAmerica, it is obvious which sites are interior, and if you take your shot at one of these walk-up sites, the campground map clearly delineates if you will have water access.

The pond, shaped like an ink stain, is large, but there are restrictions on motor size. Motors of more than 25 horsepower are prohibited, and the majority of vessels are canoes and kayaks, including rentals available near the boat launch. There is some privately owned land on Rollins, but that does not spoil the lovely views. For even quieter paddling, drop your boat in the smaller Whey Pond, located across the road at the southern end of the campground. No motorboats are permitted on Whey, making it a peaceful place to fish for brook and rainbow trout.

A beach volleyball court located alongside the shower house may keep some amused, but for most activities on dry land, you will have to travel outside the campground. At site 257, the Otter Hollow Loop trailhead set outs for 1.6 miles to Flood Passage at Floodwood Pond, and then on for almost 3 more miles to Fish Creek Pond Campground. For longer backcountry treks, hikers can follow trails in all directions to explore the St. Regis Canoe Area. Of course, this is an area best appreciated by boat, and paddlers may want to use Rollins as a staging point for longer trips.

Lake Placid and its Olympic facilities are the biggest draw for tourists in the Adirondacks, and a visit

KEY INFORMATION

ADDRESS:	Star Route Box 75 Saranac Lake, NY 12983
OPERATED BY:	New York State Department of Environmental Conservation
INFORMATION:	(518) 891-3239; www.dec.state.ny .us/website/do/ camping
OPEN:	Mid-May–early September
SITES:	287
EACH SITE HAS:	Picnic table and fire ring
ASSIGNMENT:	Choose from available sites or reservations
REGISTRATION:	On arrival or by reservation (reserve minimum 2 nights)
FACILITIES:	Water, pit and flush toilets, showers, pay phone
PARKING:	At site, maximum 2 vehicles
FEE:	$16/night
ELEVATION:	1,614 feet
RESTRICTIONS:	*Pets:* Dogs on leash with proof of currently valid rabies vaccination *Fires:* In fire rings only *Alcohol:* At site *Vehicles:* Up to 40 feet *Other:* Quiet hours 10 p.m.–7 a.m.; 25-horsepower boat-motor restriction *Reservations:* 2-night stay required

MAP

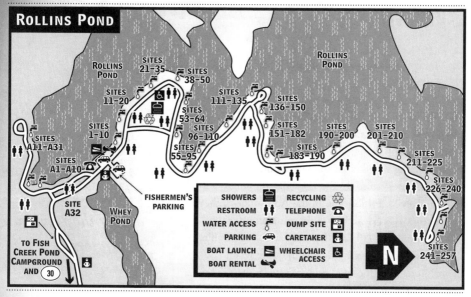

ROLLINS POND

ROLLINS POND

SITES 21-35

SITES 38-50

ROLLINS POND

ROLLINS POND

SITES 11-20

SITES 111-135

SITES 136-150

SITES 53-64

SITES 96-110

SITES 151-182

SITES 190-200

SITES 201-210

SITES 1-10

SITES A11-A31

SITES 55-95

SITES 183-190

SITES 211-225

SITES A1-A10

SITES 226-240

SITE A32

WHEY POND

FISHERMEN'S PARKING

SHOWERS		RECYCLING	
RESTROOM		TELEPHONE	
WATER ACCESS		DUMP SITE	
PARKING		CARETAKER	
BOAT LAUNCH		WHEELCHAIR ACCESS	
BOAT RENTAL			

N

SITES 241-257

TO FISH CREEK POND CAMPGROUND AND 30

GETTING THERE

From I-87, take Exit 30 to NY 73 North; follow 28 miles. In Lake Placid, take NY 86 West about 15 miles to CR 186 West, just past Saranac Lake. Go past Adirondack Regional Airport, turn left on NY 30 South, and go 9 miles to enter Fish Creek Campground. Go to Rollins Pond from site 135.

GPS COORDINATES

FISH CREEK CAMPGROUND ENTRANCE:
UTM Zone (WGS84)   18T
Easting   550991
Northing   4899396
Latitude   N 44°14'46"
Longitude   W 74°21'41"

to the top of the ski jump or a drive up Whiteface Mountain can be fun, if not exactly strenuous, activities. Tupper Lake's brand new Wild Center, a museum and miniature zoo, designed by the same people who put together Washington's Air and Space Museum, has exhibits featuring local wildlife. Saranac Lake, the closest village to the campground, is a charming place to grab a meal or do a little shopping.

So as not to be misleading, we can tell you there are definitely quieter, more remote, and more scenic facilities in the Adirondacks, but should you be lucky enough to score a waterfront site (reservations are strongly recommended), a night or two at Rollins will make for a pleasant getaway. Though this is a very large campground, its Web site describes it well: "This campground is considered by some as an overflow for Fish Creek Pond Campground, but many have discovered it to be a quiet alternative to its bigger neighbor." We assume you will not be trading in your Kelty, Marmot, or North Face gear any time soon for a rolling home with a bit of horsepower. As long as Rollins does not trade in its wonderful location and its lovely waters, we will forgive it the occasional crowded weekend.

WHAT IS THE OLDEST PUBLIC campground in the state? It depends on whom you ask. The debate still rages (for lack of a better word) among workers for the Department of Environmental Conservation. In the Catskills, they may tell you it's Devil's Tombstone. In the Adirondacks, they're likely to say it's Sacandaga. It became an official campground in 1920, but the area had been popular for years with passers-by during the time when large stretches of the road did not offer motels. The campground borders the Sacandaga River at the point where its west branch splits off; it is no wonder locals call the area "The Forks."

With so many campgrounds in the state located on lakes, it is refreshing to find one on a river. Mind you, this is not one of the wider parts of the Hudson. Although plenty of people will enjoy plopping an inner-tube into the river's little patches of white water, kayakers and canoeists will be disappointed to know that the campground doesn't even have a car-top boat launch, much less a launch for trailered boats. And when summer comes, the water often dries up, exposing the rocky riverbed. If you have a motorboat, you are better off driving south to where the river empties into Great Sacandaga Lake, a truly impressive reservoir with enough water—nearly 300 billion gallons—to go around. The lake was created in 1930 when the Sacandaga River was dammed to prevent flooding in the region.

There is also no swimming at the Sacandaga campground. In the 1970s, the Department of Environmental Conservation removed the small dam that collected water on the river and maintained a small beach. This is hardly a tragic loss. There are plenty of beaches within driving distance. Sacandaga remains an attractive campground precisely because it does

> *Campers can be lulled to sleep by the sound of rushing water rather than humming generators.*

RATINGS

Beauty: ✿ ✿ ✿ ✿
Privacy: ✿ ✿ ✿
Quiet: ✿ ✿ ✿ ✿
Cleanliness: ✿ ✿ ✿ ✿
Security: ✿ ✿ ✿ ✿
Spaciousness: ✿ ✿ ✿

not cater to day-trippers and RVs full of sunbathers. In sites along the river's edge, campers can be lulled to sleep by the sound of rushing water rather than by humming generators. And since the campground rarely reaches capacity, you do not have to reserve the best sites months in advance.

As you enter the campground, it may not seem promising. Sites 1 through 6 sit along the river but are crowded together and poorly shaded. Sites 7 through 60 lie under tall fir trees, but are even more closely packed and, except for 40 through 44, are essentially out in the open. Better suited for RVs than tents, these sites were completely empty when we visited, and for good reason. This is essentially an overflow area, and you should not bother making reservations for them.

Instead, choose something at either "The Island" or "The Berry Patch." Named by the campground staff years ago, The Island (sites 61 through 119) is located at the fork of the Sacandaga and its west branch. A sturdy, narrow bridge over the river leads to these sites from the day-use area at the northern end of the campground. Many are tempted to book sites 62 or 64, and these are certainly good choices. Tent campers wishing more room, however, may opt for sites 96 or 97, which are in the northwest corner of the campground—these require parking along the road and walking about 20 to 30 yards down to spacious clearings along the West Branch. In general, we found the sites along the West Branch to be the most desirable, but any site along the water will make for an enjoyable stay. Interior sites are well shaded by a mix of firs and hardwoods and provide easy access to the two comfort stations—but they are no different from the typical site you may find in the region.

The Berry Patch (sites 120 through 144) was named for all the wild berries that grow on the southern end of the campground. In the past, the berries have also been known to attract a black bear or two. As in most parts of the Adirondacks, bears are a concern here, and you should heed the campgrounds precautions—but it is unlikely that you will ever see one. The Berry Patch should be a little quieter than The Island. Under the shade of tall fir trees, it is a scenic

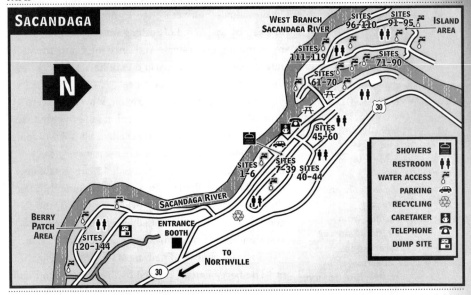

patch of sites, but the spaces themselves are a bit more jumbled together. The best of the bunch is 123, which is spacious and well situated along the river.

Even though so many sites provide easy access to the riverbank, swimming is at your own risk. Anglers come for the trout (brook, brown, and rainbow). Families with kids will appreciate the campground's Junior Naturalist program. Although no trails depart directly from the campground, the 133-mile Northville–Placid Trail has a terminus along Route 30, on the western end of a bridge over the Sacandaga. For 10 miles, the trail follows Route 30, a major road running north–south through the Adirondacks, and only those trying to complete all 133 miles feel the need to hike this section. If you are looking for an easy day hike, try the 3-mile round-trip trek to Auger Falls, located off Route 30, 10 miles north of the campground.

Quiet, safe, and easily accessible, Sacandaga has been a family favorite for generations. Many retirees have been coming to the campground since they were children. They return every year, some even staying the entire summer, shuffling spots once every two weeks. If that is not an endorsement, we don't know what is.

GETTING THERE

From I-90 (New York State Thruway), take Exit 27, Amsterdam, to NY 30 North. Follow NY 30 North for approximately 40 miles. Campground is on the left.

GPS COORDINATES

PARK ENTRANCE:
UTM Zone (WGS84) 18T
Easting 558142
Northing 4800694
Latitude N 43°21'25"
Longitude W 74°16'57"

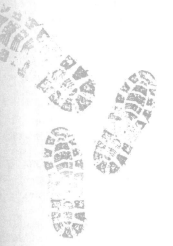

> *Even those who do not always plan ahead could be rewarded with solitude.*

IT IS SAID THAT IN THE LANGUAGE of the Iroquois Indians, *Saranac* means "cluster of stars." These days the word Saranac conjures different feelings in most New Yorkers. Nearly every grocery and convenience store in the state stocks brews made by Saranac Beer, known for its ales, lagers, and stouts. Brewed by Matt Brewing Company in the city of Utica, the beverages are made, as the Web site claims, from "the pure water that flows from the Adirondacks and the grains that grow in its unspoiled soil." Saranac Lakes, a charming village west of Lake Placid, does nothing to sully the brewery's reputation. Its three lakes (Upper, Middle, and Lower) are among the mountains' most beautiful.

Campers who own boats or are willing to spend a little money on a rental should put this book down now and reserve a campsite on Lower or Middle Saranac lakes. With 87 primitive sites (including 5 lean-tos) to choose from along the shores and on the islands of the two lakes, you are guaranteed an unforgettable Adirondack camping experience. We explored the lakes in our $100 inflatable kayak, which we would hesitate to take out on the choppy waters of, say, Lake George. It was perfect for these beauties, and after a good paddle we were greeted by an inviting campsite upon a ridge overlooking Hatchet Island.

Meticulous planners will make their summer weekend reservations nine months in advance for a place on an island, especially islands that house only one site, such as Green (13), Coal Pit (22), Larom (23), Partridge (24), Goose (27), Duck (28), Hocum Point (35), Shaw (71), Norway (74), Bartlett (75), Halfway (77), and Tick (84). As desirable as these sites are, they are not that different from shoreline sites. The wilderness is thick, there are no hiking trails, and development is prohibited on both Lower and Middle Saranac lakes. Consequently, every site is isolated, and when

RATINGS

Beauty: ✿ ✿ ✿ ✿ ✿
Privacy: ✿ ✿ ✿ ✿ ✿
Quiet: ✿ ✿ ✿ ✿ ✿
Cleanliness: ✿ ✿ ✿ ✿
Security: ✿ ✿ ✿ ✿
Spaciousness: ✿ ✿ ✿ ✿ ✿

the sun sets, campers along the shorelines may as well be on an island.

The majority of sites are located on Lower Saranac Lake (1 through 62), and all are easily reached by motorboat. Paddlers will have to do a little work to get out to the Narrows and Loon Bay on the west side of the lake. Arrive early if you plan to camp at sites 45 through 47, especially if you need to make multiple trips to ferry your supplies. Lower Saranac can be accessed from the State Bridge Boat Launch along NY 3. Boaters put in at Second Pond, where only site 62 is found. For all other sites, campers must make their way under the State Bridge (NY 3) and into First Pond, also home to just one site, number 61. Others must follow the channel markers through a narrow passage to the southern end of Lower Saranac and the rest of the sites on the lake.

A campground map is needed to find all the sites. The scale of the lake can be overwhelming, and with many bays and islands to explore, it is easy to get confused. Signs designating sites are not always easy to see, especially in the evening. A less popular car-top boat launch and a comfort station are on the eastern end of the lake in Ampersand Bay. Day visitors often use this launch to access Eagle Island (sites 1 through 5), designated as a day-use area for picnickers.

The sites on Middle Saranac Lake (63 through 87) are even more remote and therefore attract more campers with canoes or kayaks looking for quiet. Although the development of the campground at Lower Saranac officially began in 1934, the sites on Middle Saranac were not added until 1992. The lake remains an unspoiled delight, with beaches and dunes along the shoreline. It is possible to launch a boat from State Bridge and enter Middle Saranac through Kelly Slough on the western end of Lower Saranac. Traveling this way, you navigate the Saranac River and pass through a set of hand-operated locks, a lovely trip if you are not in a rush. If time is a factor, drive 4 miles west along Route 3 from State Bridge to a parking lot and put in at South Creek on the southern end of Middle Saranac.

On the northern end of Middle Saranac, tiny Weller Pond is a haven for paddlers with tents. Motor-boats turn back at the narrow passage leading to sites

KEY INFORMATION

ADDRESS:	58 Bayside Drive Saranac Lake, NY 12983
OPERATED BY:	New York State Department of Environmental Conservation
INFORMATION:	(518) 891-3170; www.dec.state.ny .us/website/do/ camping
OPEN:	Mid-May–early September
SITES:	87
EACH SITE HAS:	Picnic table and fire ring
ASSIGNMENT:	Choose from available sites or reservations
REGISTRATION:	On arrival or by reservation
FACILITIES:	Pit toilets
PARKING:	Limited at State Bridge boat launch, near regis-tration booth
FEE:	$18/night
ELEVATION:	1,541 feet
RESTRICTIONS:	*Pets:* Dogs on leash with proof of cur-rently valid rabies vaccination *Fires:* In fire rings only *Alcohol:* At site *Vehicles:* All sites are boat-access-only *Other:* Quiet hours 10 p.m.–7 a.m.; carry out all trash *Reservations:* 1-night stay allowed

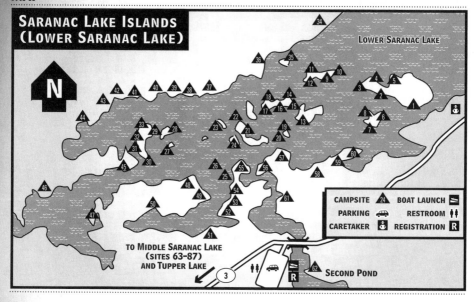

Saranac Lake Islands (Lower Saranac Lake)

GETTING THERE

From I-87 (Adirondack Northway), take Exit 30 to NY 73 North. Follow NY 73 North for 28 miles. In Lake Placid, take NY 86 West 9 miles to the village of Saranac Lake. In Saranac Lake, take NY 3 West 6 miles to the State Bridge Boat Launch on your left.

GPS COORDINATES

STATE BRIDGE BOAT LAUNCH:
UTM Zone (WGS84) 18T
Easting   564996
Northing 4904198
Latitude   N 44°17'17"
Longitude W 74°11'07"

83 through 87, so this is by far the quietest corner of the campground. Site 87 includes a lean-to, and people tend to reserve it first.

Although many stay here for the full two weeks allowed, others use the campground as a launching pad for longer trips. From Lower Saranac and Second Pond, the Saranac River runs through another set of locks and into Oseetah Lake and Lake Flower, which borders the village of Saranac Lakes. From Weller Pond, a portage of about a mile will bring you to Saginaw Bay on the northern end of Upper Saranac Lake. Or a paddle through Bartletts Carry on the southwestern end of Middle Saranac will bring you to the southeastern end of Upper Saranac. The campground doesn't include Upper Saranac because it is open for private development, but it is a magnificent, hourglass-shaped lake that makes up the southern end of the celebrated St. Regis Canoe Area. For a true adventure, the Northern Forest Canoe Trail, which has a terminus in Old Forge, runs through each of the Saranac Lakes and all the way to Fort Kent in Maine. This 740-mile trip awaits experienced, strong-shouldered paddlers and is often referred to as the water version of the Appalachian Trail.

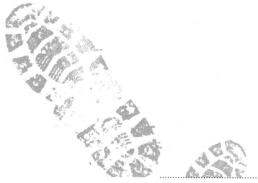

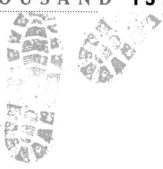

THOUSAND ISLANDS

41
MARY ISLAND
STATE PARK

ALONG THE NORTHERN BORDER of New York runs the St. Lawrence River, which flows from Lake Ontario through Canada and finally empties into the Atlantic Ocean. As the river flows more than 800 miles to the Atlantic Ocean, it passes a 50-mile stretch filled with more than 1,800 islands. These range from roughly 48 square miles to several square feet and, along with more than 3,000 shoals, make the river a veritable maze. Navigating this maze are Jet Skis, powerboats, sailboats, cruise boats, yachts, and even ocean liners, though these behemoths remain within the shipping lanes. Nestled within this maze is Mary Island, a heavily wooded 12 acres that offer the ideal setting in which to enjoy the beauty of the St. Lawrence.

The 12 sites on the island vary widely in size, views, and proximity to the access trails, numerous docks, and each other. The island is oblong, with its main axis running from southwest, where the park office and day-use area are located, to the northeast, a very short distance to Canadian waters. Most campers will approach the island from the southwest and initially encounter a service dock, public dock, and a floating campers' dock. You will want to use the middle public dock to register and then move your boat either to the neighboring floating dock for sites 1 through 5, to the northeast floating dock for sites 9 through 12, or to the sheltered fixed dock on the northeast shore for sites 6 through 10 (sites 9 and 10 are about equidistant from both northern docks). Alternatively, you can dock at the southeastern tip and access the sites along the central trail or the western trail, though this last trail runs precariously close to some cliffs. The sole comfort station is located roughly in the center of the southeastern half of the island, but it is a short distance to any of the sites.

Site 1 is closest to the office and picnic area, along the eastern edge of the island's southern tip. Although

> *Mary Island's heavily wooded 12 acres offer the ideal setting in which to enjoy the beauty of the St. Lawrence River.*

RATINGS

Beauty: ☆ ☆ ☆ ☆ ☆
Privacy: ☆ ☆ ☆ ☆
Quiet: ☆ ☆ ☆ ☆
Cleanliness: ☆ ☆
Security: ☆ ☆ ☆ ☆ ☆ ☆
Spaciousness: ☆ ☆ ☆ ☆ ☆

ADDRESS: c/o Keewaydin State Park
46165 NY 12
Alexandria Bay, NY 13607

OPERATED BY: New York State Office of Parks, Recreation and Historic Preservation

INFORMATION: (315) 654-2522; nysparks.state.ny.us

OPEN: Memorial Day–Labor Day

SITES: 12 tent sites

EACH SITE HAS: Picnic table, stand-up grill, and fire ring

ASSIGNMENT: Choose from available sites or reservations

REGISTRATION: 3 p.m.–9 p.m.

FACILITIES: Picnic areas, potable water, flush toilets, docks, showers

PARKING: At Keewaydin State Park

FEE: $13/night most tent sites; add $3/night Friday, Saturday, and holidays

ELEVATION: 241 feet

RESTRICTIONS: *Pets:* Dogs on leash with proof of currently valid rabies vaccination
Fires: In fire rings only
Alcohol: Allowed
Vehicles: All sites are boat-access only
Other: Quiet hours 10 p.m.–7 a.m.; 6 people maximum/site; maximum 14-night stay
Reservations: 2-night stay required

it has great views of the St. Lawrence, campers should be aware that the path to sites 2 through 4 passes through the site. The latter three sites lie among large, exposed slabs of granite and are closely clustered together. Site 2, although exposed, is closest to water and the southeastern campers' dock. Sites 3 and 4 are set back from the shore and have ample shade from cedars, pines, and hardwoods. Considering the proximity of these sites to each other, this area would serve groups better than campers seeking a more solitary experience.

Site 5, which is very spacious, is also on the southern tip but lies on the western shore and is consequently farther from any of the campers' docks. This site is heavily shaded by pines and cedars but has hardly any view of the river because of trees and a small electric-transfer building.

Near site 5 begins the western trail, which you could use to access site 6. However, this portion of the trail passes the precarious cliffs and site 6 can be easily reached from the main trail or the other docks. Site 6 sits high along the western cliffs but they are less precarious here, and the elevation provides expansive views of the river. A thick canopy of pines shades the spacious site, but exposed roots limit the places to pitch a tent.

Site 7 is centrally located and has direct access to the northwest fixed dock. Atop a heavily forested hill, the site offers good views of the river through the surrounding trees. There is lots of room to spread out and numerous places to pitch a tent. A short distance north from the docks lies site 8, which is undoubtedly the most spacious site on the island. Tall hardwoods shade the area, and numerous patches of grass make ideal places to pitch a tent. The site is also enhanced by great views of the river, though multiple trails serving the next two sites pass either through or very near the site.

At the very northern tip of the island lies site 9, which is one of the most scenic and secluded sites. With panoramic views of the river in three directions, it is hard to not look out to the St. Lawrence. The rugged terrain features exposed bedrock and twisted trees with ample room to spread out on grassy patches of ground. Although some spots are very close to the water, we

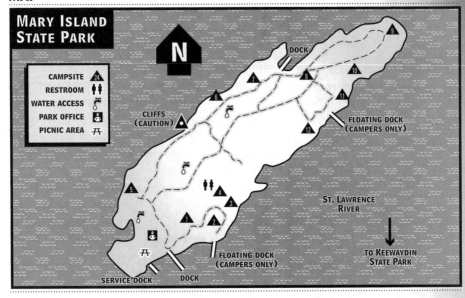

suspect campers will seek shelter rather than closeness to the water. The wind gusts strongly here, and going fishing for your tent will ruin any trip.

Traveling south along the eastern edge, campers find another great choice at site 10. Sitting atop a small hill, and with plenty of shade from the mixed hardwoods, the site offers views of the river to the east and west, along with plenty of room—large, grassy areas intermingle with exposed bedrock.

The island's remaining two sites are on its northeastern edge near the other floating campers' dock. Site 11 is closest to the dock. Since this site is on the riverbank, there is little shade, but grassy areas offer ample space to set up a tent. Site 12 has several advantages over site 11—it is more spacious, better shaded, and more remote-feeling. Both sites have spectacular views.

Although Mary Island is a stone's throw from the tip of Wellesley Island, the latter area is private. Consequently, the best access point is Keewaydin State Park on the mainland, about 2 miles away from Mary Island. Campers can park vehicles and rent small motorboats here, making Mary Island one of the most convenient boat-only sites in New York.

GETTING THERE

To Keewaydin State Park:

From Interstate 81 North, take Exit 50N, NY 12/ Alexandria Bay. Continue on NY 12 for 3.2 miles; the park entrance is on the left.

GPS COORDINATES

PARK ENTRANCE:

UTM Zone (WGS84) 18T
Easting 425677
Northing 4908127
Latitude N 44°21'56"
Longitude W 75°55'56"

SOUTH DOCK:

UTM Zone (WGS84) 18T
Easting 426591
Northing 4912878
Latitude N 44°21'56"
Longitude W 75°55'17"

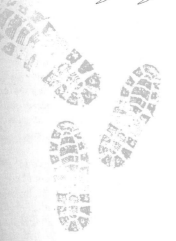

> *The campground at Wellesley Island State Park runs the whole gamut of sites, ranging from full hookups to secluded walk-ins along the river.*

THE **THOUSAND ISLANDS REGION** is a boater's haven where you can find excellent fishing and unlimited cruising opportunities. Numerous parks and public launches in the region give access to beautiful waters, but the 2,636-acre Wellesley Island State Park also offers many more recreational opportunities. Located on the northwest edge of Wellesley Island, the park has miles of hiking trails, a sandy swimming beach, a nature center, a golf course, numerous playgrounds and playfields, several boat launches, a recreation center, and a variety of habitats that provide excellent wildlife viewing. The island can be reached by boat or by driving over the first section of the multiple-span Thousand Islands Bridge, which from the north side of the island crosses the U.S.-Canada border.

The campground at Wellesley Island State Park runs the whole gamut of sites, ranging from full hookups to secluded walk-ins along the river. Tent campers should simply ignore Loops H and F as well as Area C, which are clearly for large RVs. Instead, they should try to find sites in the remaining areas (A, B, D, and E), although the type and quality of sites vary widely in these areas as well.

Most sites along Area E are lawn sites that border the surrounding forest. Although most sites on this loop won't please campers seeking beauty and solitude, there are exceptions. One such area (sites 52 through 56 as well as walk-in site 101) is accessed along a rough spur road—the area juts out into the river slightly, and this provides beautiful views. Large protrusions of bedrock and wind-swept trees add some privacy while shading the area. However, these small sites are close together and have limited parking. A similar setting exists for sites 61 through 64 and 66, which share access from a short driveway. Another

RATINGS

Beauty: ✿ ✿ ✿ ✿
Privacy: ✿ ✿ ✿
Quiet: ✿ ✿
Cleanliness: ✿ ✿ ✿
Security: ✿ ✿ ✿
Spaciousness: ✿ ✿

group of sites, 75 through 80, has views of the river, although the view is mostly of a boat launch and docks.

Area A's layout is a mishmash of loops, spurs, and switchbacks, which could make finding your site an adventure. Generally, the sites are grassy, with a few large shade trees along the edges or intermixed. With the exception of sites 17 through 30, which lie along a hillside with few flat spaces, most sites are spacious. Of particular interest are the wonderful vistas from riverside sites 44 through 49, which are shielded from the rest of the area by a hill and feel more isolated. These sites are shallow, close together, and dense with trees, precluding large trailers or RVs. A similar group of shady sites (56, 58, and 60 through 62) lies ahead on the road. This group has views of the river, but, lacking a hill, is not as private.

As with Area A, Area D has some sites that are grassy with few shade trees. The sites here are well sized, except for sites 1 through 7, which are particularly small and public. The prime sites (9 through 12, 14, 15, 19, and 20) have stunning views of the river, shade, and privacy. Although these sites are definitely a good choice, tent campers should also consider the excellent walk-in sites, 26 through 28. Access and parking for these sites is located beyond site 29, down a hill toward Area B, and on a lawn to the right. A very short walk over a small hill to the riverbank reveals spacious, shady sites with panoramic views of the river.

Whereas most areas here have only a few gems mixed with a majority of less-desirable sites, Area B is just the opposite. The entire area feels secluded, and sites seem to grow out of the woods rather than encircle large communal lawns. In general, the sites on the river side of the road are hidden away among the trees, while those on the opposite side are visible from the road and lack views. When making reservations, campers should be aware that sites 26 through 32 are electric and intended for RVs. Also, a high-traffic area exists at the end of the area where areas B and C come together and exit through Area A.

Those disclaimers aside, the campground's designated prime sites (1, 2, 6 through 8, 14 through 23, 34 through 39, and 42) are excellent, have sufficient

ADDRESS:	44927 Cross Island Road Fineview, NY 13640
OPERATED BY:	New York State Office of Parks, Recreation and Historic Preservation
INFORMATION:	(315) 482-2722; nysparks.state.ny.us
OPEN:	Late April–mid October
SITES:	435 tent sites, 115 electric sites, 57 with full hookups
EACH SITE HAS:	Picnic table and fire ring
ASSIGNMENT:	Choose from available sites or reservations
REGISTRATION:	3 p.m.–9 p.m.
FACILITIES:	Picnic areas, potable water, flush toilets, boat launch, showers, marina, 9-hole golf course
PARKING:	At site or in designated area near carry-in sites
FEE:	$13/night most tent sites; add $3/night Friday, Saturday, and holidays
ELEVATION:	253 feet
RESTRICTIONS:	*Pets:* Dogs on leash with proof of currently valid rabies vaccination *Fires:* In fire rings only *Alcohol:* Allowed *Vehicles:* RVs limited to specific sites *Other:* Quiet hours 10 p.m.–7 a.m.; 6 people maximum/site; maximum 14-night stay *Reservations:* 2-night stay required

MAP

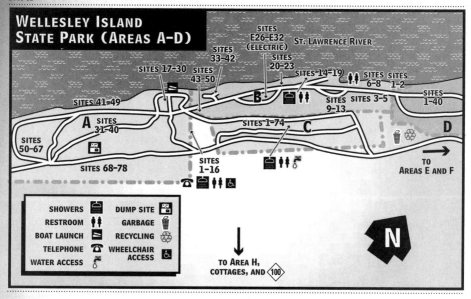

WELLESLEY ISLAND STATE PARK (AREAS A–D)

SITES E26–E32 (ELECTRIC)
ST. LAWRENCE RIVER
SITES 33–42
SITES 20–23
SITES 17–30
SITES 43–50
SITES 14–19
SITES 6–8
SITES 1–2
SITES 41–49
B
SITES 3–5
SITES 1–40
SITES 9–13
A SITES 31–40
SITES 1–74
C
D
SITES 50–67
SITES 1–16
SITES 68–78
TO AREAS E AND F

N

SHOWERS
RESTROOM
BOAT LAUNCH
TELEPHONE
WATER ACCESS
DUMP SITE
GARBAGE
RECYCLING
WHEELCHAIR ACCESS

TO AREA H, COTTAGES, AND ⟨100⟩

GETTING THERE

From I-81 North, cross over the Thousand Islands Bridge and take Exit 51, Island Road/Island Parks. Turn right on CR 191 and follow for 0.5 miles. Turn right on Thousand Islands Park Road/CR 100. After 0.5 miles, turn right on Cross Island Road and follow to the park entrance.

GPS COORDINATES

PARK ENTRANCE:

UTM Zone (WGS84)   18T
Easting   418592
Northing   4907552
Latitude   N 44°19'00"
Longitude   W 76°01'15"

space, ample shade, and exceptional views of the river. Sites 1 and 2 share access and lie downhill from the road where it climbs toward the rest of the area. Consequently, these sites feel more remote and are a great choice, since they lie directly on the riverfront. Access to sites 6 though 8 is via a rugged dirt road with blind corners that makes a steep descent toward the river and has no turnaround: you may want to walk this spur road to plan your entrance and exit. Site 8 sits above the river and closer to the main road, whereas sites 6 and 7 are right on the riverbank and basically blend together. A little farther is a grassy parking area for walk-in sites (14 through 19)—campers must climb over a steep wooded knoll to access their sites. Situated above the St. Lawrence River on a granite outcrop, these sites are a retreat from the bustle of the rest of the campground. The remaining prime sites (20 through 23, 34 through 39, and 42) are right on the riverbank, grouped in bunches of twos and threes, and reached by rough, narrow roads.

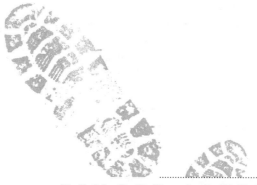
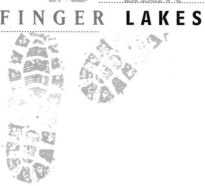

FINGER LAKES

43

BUTTERMILK FALLS STATE PARK

ON THE VERY EDGE OF ITHACA'S southern boundary lies a multiuse park that offers a special opportunity for campers wishing to visit this unique Finger Lake city. The idea of a campground practically inside a city may seem strange to some, but not if you know Ithaca. Located on the southern tip of Cayuga Lake, Ithaca presents outdoor enthusiasts with numerous activities as well as access to a wide variety of restaurants, bustling nightlife, and nearby wine trails. Ithaca seems to be surrounded by nature—in fact, there are four state parks along with numerous city- and university-managed parks within the immediate vicinity. Given the wide variety of outdoor activities available here, Buttermilk Falls State Park serves as an ideal base to explore the region.

The park includes a gorge that surrounds Buttermilk Creek, Lake Treman, and a wetland. Each of these natural features can be explored along short hiking trails, though the gorge is the park's most astounding natural feature and obviously its most popular attraction. The gorge and its striking, deep pools were dramatically carved by Buttermilk Creek, which drops from 1,000 feet to 400 feet above sea level. The water's sculpting power is particularly evident at Pinnacle Rock, a tall spire near the end of the Gorge Trail. This trail, as you might suspect, winds through the gorge, often sharing the creek bed and taking you past stone walls and up stone staircases. The stone work, originally built by the Civilian Conservation Corps during the Depression, provides an interesting comparison of man's and nature's work on the local stone. At Buttermilk Falls, the creek cascades white and frothy across a wide rock face and tumbles to a pool below. At the base of this waterfall is a small but deep swimming area that is accessible by the park's lower entrance and main parking lot.

> *The idea of a campground practically inside a city may seem strange to some, but not if you know Ithaca.*

RATINGS

Beauty: ✿ ✿
Privacy: ✿ ✿ ✿
Quiet: ✿ ✿ ✿
Cleanliness: ✿ ✿ ✿
Security: ✿ ✿ ✿
Spaciousness: ✿ ✿

ADDRESS: NY 13
Ithaca, NY 14850

OPERATED BY: New York State
Office of Parks,
Recreation and His-
toric Preservation

INFORMATION: (607) 273-5761;
nysparks.state.ny.us

OPEN: Mid-May–
mid-October

SITES: 46

EACH SITE HAS: Picnic table and
fire ring

ASSIGNMENT: Choose from
available sites or
reservations

REGISTRATION: 3 p.m.–9 p.m.

FACILITIES: Picnic areas, pavilions, playground,
swimming area,
bathhouse, potable
water, flush toilets,
showers

PARKING: At site

FEE: $13/night

ELEVATION: 410 feet

RESTRICTIONS: *Pets:* Dogs on leash
with proof of cur-
rently valid rabies
vaccination
Fires: In fire rings
only
Alcohol: Prohibited in
swimming area
Vehicles: RVs and
trailers allowed
Other: Quiet hours
10 p.m.–7 a.m.; 6
people maximum/
site; maximum
14-night stay
Reservations: 2-night
stay required

The park's campground is accessed from this same parking area and is separated from the rest of the park by a long, winding paved road that climbs a steep hillside. The camping area, which begins with a handful of rental cabins, is laid out in a single loop with a short spur road containing four more tent sites. All of the sites, which are mostly dirt with some grassy spots, are shaded by a canopy of mixed hardwood trees. There is not much understory, so the sites are visible to each other. But they're amply spaced, and changes in elevation between the eastern and western edges of the area prevent it from feeling crowded.

The sites along the western edge lie near a drop-off and have less space then those on the interior of the loop. Sites on the eastern outer edge are the most desirable: they are spacious, more private, and border the surrounding woods. The most private sites are the four situated along a short spur road at the end of the campground loop.

Campers who can't find a site at Buttermilk Falls can drive south a little over 1 mile to Robert H. Treman State Park, where there are considerably more campsites. However, the sites here are mostly situated on a grassy field and offer little in the way of shade and privacy. From this state park, adventurers can hike along Enfield Creek and its related gorge, which has waterfalls and water-sculpted rocks.

Fillmore Glen State Park, a short drive north of Ithaca, offers more hiking trails in another dramatic gorge. Camping is available here as well, though the sites here are even more crowded and less private than the ones at Robert H. Treman State Park.

Boaters wishing to gain access to Cayuga Lake can drive north from Buttermilk Falls State Park a few miles to Allan H. Treman State Marine Park, where there is a boat launch, or about 15 miles farther to Taughannock Falls State Park (see its description on page 159). Since access to one state park grants vehicle access to others on the same day, take the time to explore the trails and gorges at these other parks as well. After all, as the saying goes, "Ithaca is Gorges."

MAP

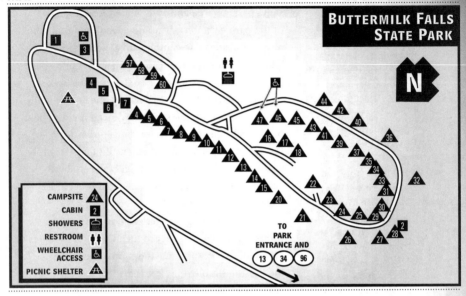

BUTTERMILK FALLS STATE PARK

N

CAMPSITE	24
CABIN	2
SHOWERS	
RESTROOM	
WHEELCHAIR ACCESS	
PICNIC SHELTER	

TO
PARK
ENTRANCE AND
13 34 96

GETTING THERE

From Interstate 81 South, take Exit 12, NY 281/Cortland. Stay left on off-ramp until you reach stop sign. Turn left onto NY 281; follow 3.8 miles. NY 281 becomes NY 13; continue on NY 13 through Dryden into Ithaca. After passing NY 79/Main Street, continue 2 miles. Park entrance is on the left.

GPS COORDINATES

PARK ENTRANCE:

UTM Zone (WGS84)	18T
Easting	374796
Northing	4697212
Latitude	N 42°25'02"
Longitude	W 76°31'18"

Bluff Point

44
KEUKA LAKE
STATE PARK

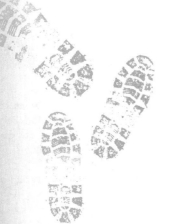

> *Shaped like a Y, Keuka Lake is sometimes called Crooked Lake.*

ABIRD'S-EYE VIEW OF WESTERN NEW YORK reveals 11 narrow lakes, each of which runs roughly north–south. Their unusual likenesses to fingers on a hand obviously led to their name, the Finger Lakes. Keuka Lake is the only lake among the 11 that is not perfectly linear in shape: it is shaped like a Y and so is sometimes called Crooked Lake. Further, the lake is distinct from its neighbors in that it is also the only one that drains into another of the Finger Lakes— in this case, into Seneca Lake by way of Keuka Lake Outlet. At one time, this outlet was transformed into a canal that connected the two lakes, but it was eventually abandoned as a canal in 1877. Aside from these characteristics, it shares all of the other familiar traits of a Finger Lake in that it is glacially formed, is very deep, has it own wine trail, and is an ideal place to go fishing or boating. Incidentally, *Keuka* comes from the Iroquois word *kyoo-ka,* which means "canoe landing."

The campground at Keuka Lake is uphill from the park entrance. It is laid out in three large, one-way loops: Deer Run, Twin Fawns, and Esperanza View. The sites are spacious, open to the sky, grassy, and spread out along the loops. Additionally, the center of each loop is dense with conifers, which effectively divide the loop into smaller, private sections. Most sites have a shade tree as well as shrubs and thick vegetation, which increases privacy. The sites are large enough for a camping area, vehicles, and a small boat trailer. Considering that the lake is the park's main feature, space for a boat is a great benefit. Each loop is served with its own comfort station and playground. Dumpsters and recycling stations are situated along the access road.

The Deer Run Loop (sites 51 through 100) is a little less private than the other loops, but has many good sites. None of the sites in this loop contain

RATINGS

Beauty: ✿ ✿
Privacy: ✿ ✿ ✿ ✿
Quiet: ✿ ✿ ✿
Cleanliness: ✿ ✿ ✿ ✿
Security: ✿ ✿ ✿
Spaciousness: ✿ ✿ ✿ ✿ ✿

electric hookups. The best sites are along the beginning of the loop, on the eastern edge and interior.
These sites have dense shrubs and grasses as well as
large shade trees. Where the loop turns back toward
the entrance, the sites become more open, with less
shade and vegetation, making them less private. Near
the loop's entrance, the sites become wide open,
with no shade and only sparse vegetation. The exterior
sites are clearly visible from the access road; the
interior sites have direct access to the playground.

The Twin Fawns Loop (sites 1 through 50) contains
the park's most shady sites, graced as they are by very
large willows. The exterior of the loop contains the
shadiest sites as well as denser vegetation dividing the
sites. The best sites, both on the interior and exterior,
lie on the western edge of the loop and are primarily
nonelectric. Farther along the loop, the sites are quite
large and most have electric hookups. Unlike the
Deer Run Loop, all of the sites here are effectively
removed from the rest of the sites within the loop,
making them a little more desirable.

The last loop, Esperanza View (101 through 150),
consists of an upper section along its eastern edge
and a lower section on its western edge. The change in
elevation and a dense conifer center increases this
loop's overall privacy, but sites in the upper section are
far more desirable than those in the lower section.
There are fewer shade trees in the upper section, but
this permits views up and down the lake valley. Sites
in the upper section, though almost entirely electric,
offer added privacy with an additional border of
dense shrubs along the roadside. The configuration of
shrubs and trees creates the feeling of outdoor rooms.

Campers won't find as many hiking opportunities
here as at some other New York campgrounds—but
access to the lake and its related water sports is the real
attraction. The lake is the third largest of the Finger
Lakes: its width varies from 0.5 miles to 2 miles along
its 19.6-mile length. The total surface area measures
roughly 11,730 acres, and the deepest point is 183 feet.
A public boat launch is located past the park's picnic
and swimming areas and is available to anyone paying
the park entrance fee. Boating and fishing regulations

KEY INFORMATION

ADDRESS:	3370 Pepper Road Bluff Point, NY 14478
OPERATED BY:	New York State Office of Parks, Recreation and Historic Preservation
INFORMATION:	(315) 536-3666; nysparks.state.ny.us
OPEN:	End of April– end of October
SITES:	150 tent sites, 53 electric sites
EACH SITE HAS:	Picnic table and fire ring
ASSIGNMENT:	Choose from available sites or reservations
REGISTRATION:	3 p.m.–9 p.m.
FACILITIES:	Picnic areas, pavilion, potable water, flush toilets, park store, boat launch, showers
PARKING:	At site
FEE:	$13/night most tent sites; add $3/night Friday, Saturday, and holidays
ELEVATION:	817 feet
RESTRICTIONS:	*Pets:* Dogs on leash with proof of currently valid rabies vaccination *Fires:* In fire rings only *Alcohol:* Allowed *Vehicles:* RVs and trailers allowed *Other:* Quiet hours 10 p.m.–7 a.m.; 6 people maximum/ site; maximum 14-night stay *Reservations:* 2-night stay required

MAP

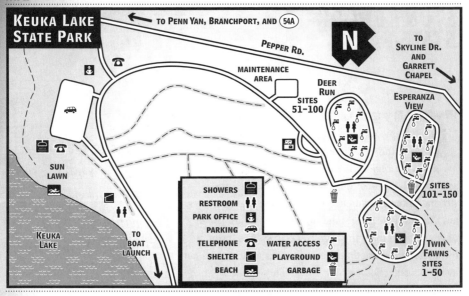

Keuka Lake State Park map with legend:
- SHOWERS
- RESTROOM
- PARK OFFICE
- PARKING
- TELEPHONE
- SHELTER
- BEACH
- WATER ACCESS
- PLAYGROUND
- GARBAGE

GETTING THERE

From I-90 (New York State Thruway), take Exit 42. Take NY 14 South through Geneva; 12.7 miles past Geneva, go right on NY 54. Turn right to stay on NY 54; go 4.5 miles to Penn Yan. Go left on NY 54/Main Street, then right on NY 54A/Elm Street. Follow 6.3 miles; go left on Pepper Road. Park entrance is on right.

GPS COORDINATES

PARK ENTRANCE:
UTM Zone (WGS84)   18T
Easting   325182
Northing   4717587
Latitude   N 42°35'27"
Longitude   W 77°07'50"

are available at the entrance and on the Web at **www.keukalakeassoc.org.** Diving, motorboats, Jet Skis, and waterskiing are all allowed, as are sailboats, kayaks, and canoes.

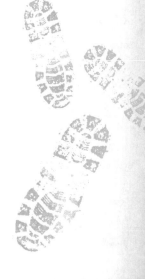

THE FINGERS LAKES REGION was shaped by
multiple periods of glaciation during the Ice
Age. Indeed, the entire state of New York,
except in the region of Allegany State Park, bears the
scars and deposits of huge sheets of ice. The most
striking of the glacial effects, besides the region's lakes,
are the dramatic gorges that formed as the last sheets
of ice receded from the region. Long swaths through
hillsides were eroded further as brooks and streams cut
away the softer sedimentary rock. These gorges can
be seen throughout the region, but no state park other
than Stony Brook allows you to camp along the water's
edge. Although Stony Brook's camping areas are not
situated within the most dramatic parts of the gorge,
there are plenty of scenic brookside sites available.

The park's campground is divided into two areas,
the first of which contains sites 1 through 53 and is
laid out as a single loop with one spur road. Large
evergreens provide ample shade throughout this area,
though the trees are densest at the exterior of the
loop and along the spur road. Along the southern edge
of the loop and spur is a steep hillside, at the bottom of
which flows a stream that feeds Stony Brook. Sites
that back up to this edge look down upon the stream
and into the surrounding forest. Sites on the loop's
interior are close together, grassy, and very public due
to proximity to this area's comfort station. The first
few sites (16 through 19) on the loop's exterior are also
grassy but very small, as they back up to a hillside that
separates them from ones on the spur road. The other
sites along the exterior of the loop are larger and have
a gravelly dirt base. The spur road rises above the loop
sites, which effectively removes sites along the spur
road (35 through 53) from the more public spaces of
this area. These sites are more densely wooded and
have a gravelly dirt base as well. Most sites along the

> *Few of the Fingers
> Lakes region's parks
> offer as scenic a
> campground as the
> one at Stony Brook.*

RATINGS

Beauty: ✪ ✪ ✪ ✪
Privacy: ✪ ✪ ✪
Quiet: ✪ ✪ ✪
Cleanliness: ✪ ✪ ✪
Security: ✪ ✪ ✪
Spaciousness: ✪ ✪ ✪

KEY INFORMATION

ADDRESS: 10820 Route 36S
Dansville, NY 14437

OPERATED BY: New York State
Office of Parks,
Recreation and His-
toric Preservation

INFORMATION: (585) 335-5530;
nysparks.state.ny.us

OPEN: April–end of
October

SITES: 125 tent sites

EACH SITE HAS: Picnic table and
fire ring

ASSIGNMENT: Choose from
available sites or
reservations

REGISTRATION: 3 p.m.–9 p.m.

FACILITIES: Picnic areas, pavilion, potable water,
flush toilets, conces-
sion stand, bath-
house, tennis courts,
playground, showers

PARKING: At site

FEE: $13/night most tent
sites; add $3/night
Friday, Saturday,
and holidays

ELEVATION: 384 feet

RESTRICTIONS: *Pets:* Dogs on leash
with proof of cur-
rently valid rabies
vaccination
Fires: In fire rings
only
Alcohol: Not allowed
in campground
Vehicles: RVs and
trailers allowed
Other: Quiet hours
10 p.m.–7 a.m.; 6
people maximum/
site; maximum
14-night stay
Reservations: 2-night
stay required

spur road are grouped in threes or fours that share narrow parking areas. This configuration makes it hard to tell where some sites begin and end. Consequently, these grouped sites are probably best suited to large camping parties—solitary campers would most likely prefer some of the other sites this park has to offer.

The second area, sites 54 though 130, is by far the largest, with some spacious sites situated along Stony Brook. Like those in the previous area, these sites are shaded by large evergreens, and the trees here are denser than those at the sites mentioned above. Similarly, these sites also have gravelly dirt bases with no shrubbery or understory. The layout includes a very small loop and a much larger loop consisting of both an upper and lower leg. Where the upper and lower legs reconnect, a short road to a public parking area begins. This layout allows the sites to feel removed from the entire campground but not from their immediate neighbors. As campers descend from the park's main road to this area and its upper leg, they will see the very small loop of congested sites (55 through 60). Near this small loop are several more shared-access sites (54, 68 through 72). Along the outer edge of the upper leg are many large sites with features similar to most other sites in this area.

Down at the lower leg, the interior sites back up to the hillside that separates the upper and lower legs, and thus have a more enclosed feel. These sites are well spaced, with some being deep and large. The first few sites (112 through 116) on the lower leg's exterior are set back from the road toward Stony Brook—these sites share the same parking area. The remaining sites along the exterior of the leg lie directly on the edge of Stony Brook, which makes these sites unique to the campground. Sites along the water's edge are not as spacious as some of the others, but there are a few gems. As you drive back up to the upper leg, you find the park's remaining sites (87 through 92)— these are very small, grassy sites wedged between the road and a steep hillside.

The park has three hiking trails, two along the gorge's rim and one along the gorge's bottom, all of which are accessible from the campground area. The

MAP

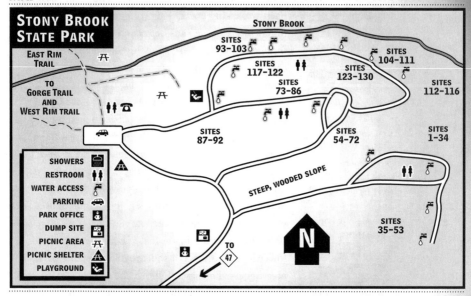

STONY BROOK STATE PARK

STONY BROOK

SITES 93–103

SITES 104–111

EAST RIM TRAIL

SITES 117–122

SITES 123–130

SITES 112–116

TO GORGE TRAIL AND WEST RIM TRAIL

SITES 73–86

SITES 87–92

SITES 54–72

SITES 1–34

STEEP, WOODED SLOPE

SITES 35–53

N

TO 47

SHOWERS
RESTROOM
WATER ACCESS
PARKING
PARK OFFICE
DUMP SITE
PICNIC AREA
PICNIC SHELTER
PLAYGROUND

three trails join at the lower end of the gorge, where a dam across the brook provides the park's swimming area. The gorge-bottom trail winds past three large waterfalls while climbing up and down stone staircases built by the Depression-era Civilian Conservation Corps, which also built most of the park's buildings. There are many beautiful gorges in the Fingers Lakes region, but few of the region's parks offer as scenic a campground as the one at Stony Brook.

GETTING THERE

From I-90 (New York State Thruway), take Exit 46, I-390 South/Corning. Follow I-390 for 43.3 miles to Exit 4, Dansville. Go right on NY 36 South. At 1.2 miles, main park entrance is on left. Stay on NY 36 a little over 1 mile and go left on CR 47. Campground entrance is on left.

GPS COORDINATES

PARK ENTRANCE:
UTM Zone (WGS84) 18T
Easting 278438
Northing 4710095
Latitude N 42°30'41"
Longitude W 77°41'49"

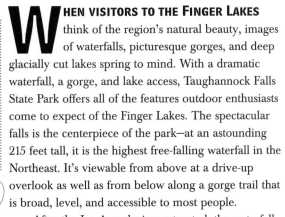

> *Taughannock Falls State Park offers all the features that outdoor enthusiasts come to expect of the Finger Lakes.*

WHEN VISITORS TO THE **FINGER LAKES** think of the region's natural beauty, images of waterfalls, picturesque gorges, and deep glacially cut lakes spring to mind. With a dramatic waterfall, a gorge, and lake access, Taughannock Falls State Park offers all of the features outdoor enthusiasts come to expect of the Finger Lakes. The spectacular falls is the centerpiece of the park—at an astounding 215 feet tall, it is the highest free-falling waterfall in the Northeast. It's viewable from above at a drive-up overlook as well as from below along a gorge trail that is broad, level, and accessible to most people.

After the Ice Age glaciers retreated, the waterfall was formed over millennia as Taughannock Creek flowed over hard Tully limestone and cut away at Sherburne sandstone and Geneseo shale. The erosion process formed a hanging canyon, so the sheer walls at the falls' basin are actually 400 feet high, which makes the basin a very dramatic vantage point. The waters surge in the spring, making the falls truly a wonder, but in summer they die down, so visitors may wish to time their trip early in the spring to see the falls in its full majesty. The rocks washed away by Taughannock Creek and over the falls have, over the centuries, formed a delta on Cayuga Lake—today the site of the park's lawn, picnic area, and most of the day-use activities. As in other New York state parks, most of the structures and other park infrastructure are products of work by park staff and the Civilian Conservation Corps during the 1930s.

The campground in Taughannock Falls State Park is located off a public road that leads to the Falls Overlook. The camping area is essentially laid out in a figure eight that runs across a steep hillside. Consequently, a change in elevation as you move around the loop helps to increase privacy throughout the campground.

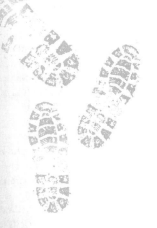

RATINGS

Beauty: ☆ ☆ ☆
Privacy: ☆ ☆ ☆
Quiet: ☆ ☆ ☆
Cleanliness: ☆ ☆ ☆
Security: ☆ ☆
Spaciousness: ☆ ☆ ☆

The sites near the entrance are electric, mostly gravel, and obviously favorable for RVs and trailers. At the next part of the figure eight, the sites are designated mostly as tent-only and have larger trees, increased shade, and a denser understory. As you drive through the upper part of the figure eight, the sites are designated as tent and trailer and are consequently very spacious, have ample shade, and some understory.

The road then descends to the lower part of the loop, where there are intermittent views of Cayuga Lake through the trees. In summer, the canopy of hardwoods downslope from the campsites obscures the view, but after the leaves drop in fall there are open views of the lake. The sites along the exterior here are large, more shaded, and definitely offer the best views in the campground. Quite a few of these sites are tent-only and blend into the large hardwood trees. The interior sites here are smaller, have less shade, are closer together, and have very limited lake views. As the loop gets closer to the entrance, the sites on both the interior and exterior get smaller and closer together, and their views of the lake are increasingly blocked by the surrounding trees.

Hiking in the park includes the gorge trail, two rim trails, and a multiuse trail. On the park's lawn are multiple picnic areas; fishing is available from the lakeshore and from the fishing pier. Cayuga Lake's fish include lake, brown, and rainbow trout; smallmouth, largemouth, and rock bass; yellow perch; chain pickerel; northern pike; and landlocked salmon. A public boat launch and marina are located south of Taughannock Creek, but the park's Web site indicates that the launch is not suitable for any type of sailboat.

Overnight berths are available by calling the park in advance. Swimming is restricted to a designated area in a protected cove on the south side of the park's lawn area. The park also offers a summer concert series, so campers might want to book their trip to coincide with a favorite performance; call for schedules. A short drive south brings campers to Ithaca and all of its attractions, and to the north and west are some of the popular Finger Lakes wine trails.

KEY INFORMATION

ADDRESS:	Taughannock Park Road Trumansburg, NY 14886
OPERATED BY:	New York State Office of Parks, Recreation and Historic Preservation
INFORMATION:	(607) 387-6739; nysparks.state.ny.us
OPEN:	Mid-May– mid-October
SITES:	76 tent sites, 16 electric sites
EACH SITE HAS:	Picnic table and fire ring
ASSIGNMENT:	Choose from available sites or reservations
REGISTRATION:	3 p.m.–9 p.m.
FACILITIES:	Picnic areas, pavilions, potable water, flush toilets, snack bar, bathhouse, marina, playgrounds, showers
PARKING:	At site
FEE:	$13/night most tent sites; add $3/night Friday, Saturday, and holidays
ELEVATION:	396 feet
RESTRICTIONS:	*Pets:* Dogs on leash with proof of currently valid rabies vaccination *Fires:* In fire rings only *Alcohol:* Allowed *Vehicles:* RVs and trailers limited to specific sites *Other:* Quiet hours 10 p.m.–7 a.m.; 6 people maximum/ site; maximum 14-night stay *Reservations:* 2-night stay required

MAP

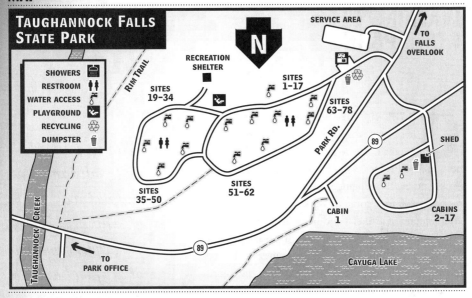

GETTING THERE

From I-81 South, take Exit 12, NY 281/Cortland. Stay left on off-ramp until stop sign. Turn left on NY 281; follow 3.8 miles. NY 281 becomes NY 13; follow through Dryden into Ithaca. Go right on West Buffalo Street/NY 89/ NY 96, then right again on NY 89; follow 9.3 miles to park entrance on right.

GPS COORDINATES

PARK ENTRANCE:

UTM Zone (WGS84)   18T
Easting   368761
Northing   4711578
Latitude   N 42°32'44"
Longitude   W 76°35'54"

47
WATKINS GLEN STATE PARK

ON THE SOUTHERN SHORES of Seneca Lake lies one of the most spectacular gorges in the Finger Lakes region. With its hand-cut tunnels, arched bridges, winding stone staircases, water-drilled pools, 19 plunging waterfalls, and water-sculpted rock, the 400-foot gorge of Watkins Glen is a wondrous combination of artificial and naturally carved beauty.

During the 19th century, the glen was operated as a tourist resort until New York state purchased this marvel in 1906. The Gorge Trail explores the interior of the gorge, and you can visit the rim via the Indian and South Rim trails. In fact, the South Rim Trail forms a part of both the Finger Lakes Trail and the North Country National Scenic Trail. The Finger Lakes Trail traverses part of southern and western New York, connecting the Catskill Mountains with Allegany State Park; the North Country National Scenic Trail, when completed, will connect Lake Champlain in New York with Lake Sakakawea in North Dakota. Less ambitious hikers or those with time constraints should hike the Gorge Trail as a round-trip, or take advantage of a park shuttle bus to return to the main parking area.

The campgroundsix "villages," or loops, are named after Native American tribes that inhabited New York: Cayuga, Mohawk, Oneida, Onondaga, Seneca, and Tuscarora. Almost all the sites are densely forested; each loop has a comfort station and multiple dumpsters.

Although Cayuga Village (sites 1 through 49) has a similar number of sites as the other loops, it is slightly smaller and consequently the sites are less spacious and closer together. Large red pines thoroughly shade the area, but there is very little understory, leaving the sites visible to each other. Even less private are the sites (odd numbers 27 through 37, and 38) that back up to Mohawk Village and the ten sites (39 through 49) situated directly on a road that serves two of the loops.

> *With its plunging waterfalls and water-sculpted rock, the gorge of Watkins Glen is a wondrous combination of artificial and natural beauty.*

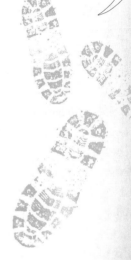

RATINGS

Beauty: ☆ ☆
Privacy: ☆ ☆ ☆
Quiet: ☆ ☆ ☆
Cleanliness: ☆ ☆ ☆
Security: ☆ ☆ ☆ ☆
Spaciousness: ☆ ☆ ☆

KEY INFORMATION

ADDRESS:	State Route 419 Watkins Glen, NY 14891
OPERATED BY:	New York State Office of Parks, Recreation and Historic Preservation
INFORMATION:	(607) 535-4511; nysparks.state.ny.us
OPEN:	May–end of October
SITES:	305 sites, 54 electric
EACH SITE HAS:	Picnic table and fire ring
ASSIGNMENT:	Choose from available sites or reservations
REGISTRATION:	3 p.m.–9 p.m.
FACILITIES:	Picnic areas, pavilion, potable water, flush toilets, park store, swimming pool, showers
PARKING:	At site
FEE:	$13 (Oneida Village) $17/night most other tent sites; add $3/ night Friday, Saturday, and holidays
ELEVATION:	726 feet
RESTRICTIONS:	*Pets:* Dogs on leash with proof of currently valid rabies vaccination *Fires:* In fire rings only *Alcohol:* Allowed *Vehicles:* RVs and trailers limited to specific sites *Other:* Quiet hours 10 p.m.–7 a.m.; 6 people maximum/ site; maximum 14-night stay *Reservations:* 2-night stay required

The neighboring loop, Mohawk Village (sites 50 through 105), contains the only electric sites in the campground, which cost more than those in other loops. The initial sites are closest to Cayuga Village, are quite large, and lie a little higher than the rest of the loop. These sites are best suited to larger RVs and contain all of the higher-amp electric sites. Near the loop's eastern edge, the road descends, providing wooded views of Seneca Lake. The change in elevation makes this area far more removed from the rest of the village—but the understory remains sparse, and the sites here are still visible to each other. Given the increased cost, tent campers might want to look elsewhere—but since these are the only views of the lake, take a peek to see what is available.

Nestled in the center of the entire campground is Oneida Village (sites 106 through 153), which, incidentally, offers the most affordable sites. A canopy of pines and hardwoods shades the area, and a dense understory and multiple changes in terrain lead to a wide variety of site sizes. Not surprisingly, most of the sites here are designated as tent-only—since the sites are considerably more private than in the previous villages, campers seeking seclusion and who don't require much space should give this area a good look.

The next two villages, Onondaga and Seneca, are off a short access road but are separate enough not to neighbor each other. Sites within Onondaga Village (154 through 203) are generally large and shady—the notable exceptions being sites 185 through 188, which lie on a lawn and are very public. The initial sites along this loop have dense saplings between them and are tent-only. The sites get larger and more spread out near the loop's midpoint, with sites along the periphery extending farthest into the surrounding forest. Seneca Village (sites 204 through 251) is similar to Onondaga, but because its loop is larger, the sites are more spread out and feel more remote. Tall hardwoods shade all of the sites here, and some understory is present throughout. A deep woodland setting generally characterizes these two loops, with plenty of good options for tent campers.

The last village, Tuscarora (sites 252 through 305), encircles a large lawn that contains a playground—but

MAP

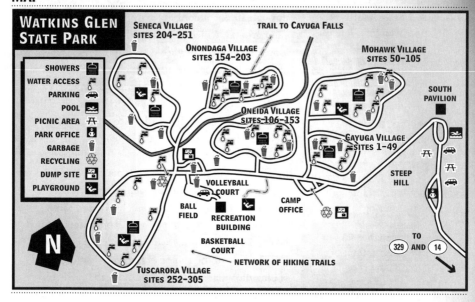

WATKINS GLEN STATE PARK

SENECA VILLAGE SITES 204–251

TRAIL TO CAYUGA FALLS

ONONDAGA VILLAGE SITES 154–203

MOHAWK VILLAGE SITES 50–105

SHOWERS
WATER ACCESS
PARKING
POOL
PICNIC AREA
PARK OFFICE
GARBAGE
RECYCLING
DUMP SITE
PLAYGROUND

SOUTH PAVILION

ONEIDA VILLAGE SITES 106–153

CAYUGA VILLAGE SITES 1–49

STEEP HILL

VOLLEYBALL COURT

BALL FIELD

RECREATION BUILDING

CAMP OFFICE

BASKETBALL COURT

TO 329 AND 14

NETWORK OF HIKING TRAILS

TUSCARORA VILLAGE SITES 252–305

N

since this loop is much larger than previous ones, the sites are more spread out. Although many sites along the interior either back up to or lie upon the lawn area, some of the park's best sites are found here. The first dozen are similar to those in Oneida Village, since they have dense undergrowth and are fairly shallow. Near site 265, interior sites sprawl into the encircled lawn and peripheral sites extend back into the forest. Sites on the perimeter are tent-only, their dense vegetation and depth providing some seclusion. Interior sites revert to a woodland setting at site 276, but beyond site 283, sites on both sides of the road open up to the lawn. The sites again revert to a woodland setting at sites 291 and 294, but these are far more closely spaced than other wooded sites in the loop. The last few lie next to the loop's entrance and consequently are not very private or desirable.

Visitors to the park should be aware that the annual Watkins Glen International NASCAR races, held each summer, results in solid bookings for a week or more at this and every other nearby campground.

GETTING THERE

From I-90 (New York State Thruway), take Exit 42, NY 14/Geneva/Lyons. Follow NY 14 south for 42.4 miles through most of the village of Watkins Glen. The main park entrance is on the right.

GPS COORDINATES

PARK ENTRANCE:

UTM Zone (WGS84)   18T
Easting   345941
Northing   4693215
Latitude   N 42°22'33"
Longitude   W 76°52'16

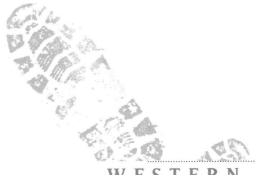

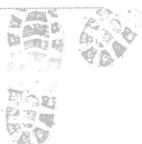

WESTERN
NEW YORK

48
ALLEGANY STATE PARK: CAIN HOLLOW (QUAKER AREA)

AT **65,000 ACRES,** Allegany State Park is the largest state park in New York. Considering that the park borders Pennsylvania's Allegheny National Forest, which covers more than 500,000 acres, this area is truly a vast wilderness. This wilderness park is unique for two reasons: first, unlike the Adirondacks and Catskills, it is a state park, not a state forest; and second, the area was unglaciated. Glacial influences on the landscape are evident across all of New York except, for all practical purposes, within the boundaries of this park. Untouched by Ice Age glaciers, the landscape, topography, and geology of Allegany State Park are quite different from what most New Yorkers are used to. This unglaciated area, called the Salamanca Reentrant, consists of more angular and rugged terrain than the deeply gouged troughs and subdued terrain found in the rest of the state. Established in 1921 to provide the western half of New York with its own "wilderness playground," the park is a great destination for campers wishing to vary their wilderness experiences in New York.

The park consists of two main sections, the Red House Area to the north and the Quaker Area to the south. Within these two sections are 375 cabins (the actual number available varies from year to year and season to season) and three camping areas: the Cain Hollow Camping Area, the Red House Tent and Trailer Area, and the Diehl Tent and Trailer Trail. Located in the Quaker Area, the Diehl campsites are intermixed with cabins and are not particularly desirable, unless part of your camping party wishes to stay in cabins. The Red House Area, with a total of 139 tent and RV sites, has a densely wooded section (Loops B through E) with sites that vary widely in size, spacing, and privacy, as well as an open field area (Loop A) containing more-public (and less-desirable) sites. Although there are

> *Untouched by Ice Age glaciers, the landscape, topography, and geology of Allegany State Park are quite different from what most New Yorkers are used to.*

RATINGS

Beauty: ✿ ✿
Privacy: ✿ ✿ ✿ ✿
Quiet: ✿ ✿ ✿
Cleanliness: ✿ ✿ ✿
Security: ✿ ✿ ✿ ✿
Spaciousness: ✿ ✿ ✿

ADDRESS: Cain Hollow Road
Salamanca, NY 14779

OPERATED BY: New York State
Office of Parks,
Recreation and His-
toric Preservation

INFORMATION: (716) 354-2182;
nysparks.state.ny.us

OPEN: Memorial Day–
Columbus Day
(Cain Hollow
Camping Area)

SITES: 164 tent sites,
94 electric sites

EACH SITE HAS: Picnic table and
fire ring

ASSIGNMENT: Choose from
available sites or
reservations

REGISTRATION: 3 p.m.–9 p.m.

FACILITIES: Picnic areas, pavilion, potable water,
flush toilets, park
store, boat launch,
museums, showers

PARKING: At site

FEE: $13/night most tent
sites; add $3/night
Friday, Saturday,
and holidays

ELEVATION: 1,453 feet

RESTRICTIONS: *Pets:* Dogs on leash
with proof of cur-
rently valid rabies
vaccination
Fires: In fire rings
only
Alcohol: Allowed
Vehicles: RVs and
trailers allowed
Other: Quiet hours
10 p.m.–7 a.m.; 6
people maximum/
site; maximum
14-night stay
Reservations: 2-night
stay required

many good sites in the Red House Area, the nonelectric sites at Cain Hollow, described below, are prime.

Also located in the Quaker Area (and sometimes referred to by that name outside the park), Cain Hollow is divided into two main groups: sites 1 through 42 and sites 43 through 164. The first group lies on an open field without any trees or privacy—but since these all have electric hookups, they are for trailers and RVs only. The second group has a central road that serves several spur roads and loops, which interweave into one another but eventually rejoin the central road. The numbering system is a bit confusing, as roads and loops seem to be bisecting each other and numbers run counterclockwise and clockwise in different sections. The only real way to figure out why you are now at site 121 after having driven past, say, site 79 is to look at a map. The entire group is on a hill, and the changes in elevation help increase the privacy throughout. Although the higher sites have partially obscured views into the sites below, the lower sites can't see into the sites above them at all. Consequently, the most private sites lie on the uppermost part of the hill. Coincidentally, these sites (140 through 164) are also among the most spacious in the group, making them the best choice for campers who wish for a little more solitude. Sites 96 through 109 and 131 through 139, on the hill's northeastern edge, are grassy and quite open, with little shade. The interior sites (74 through 95 and 120 through 130) are shady, well sized, and surrounded with brush, making them private and a good choice for most tent campers. The exceptions are sites 110 through 119, which are fairly open (and have electric hookups).

Bordering the main access road are two groups of very shady sites (most have electric hookups). Sites 43 through 55 are close together and fairly public. Sites 56 through 73 are more spread out and have a denser understory; many are by a creek. These sites are a good choice, but their electric hookups and designation as prime sites makes them more expensive.

Though most of this park can be considered wilderness, it also contains pockets of development

MAP

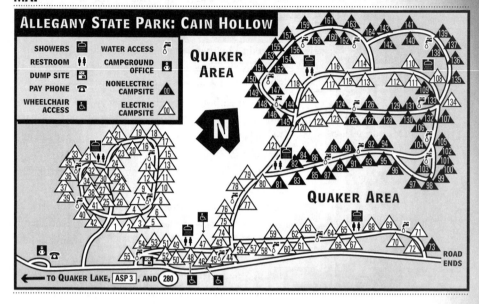

ALLEGANY STATE PARK: CAIN HOLLOW

SHOWERS		WATER ACCESS	
RESTROOM		CAMPGROUND OFFICE	
DUMP SITE		NONELECTRIC CAMPSITE	00
PAY PHONE		ELECTRIC CAMPSITE	00
WHEELCHAIR ACCESS			

QUAKER AREA

N

QUAKER AREA

ROAD ENDS

⟵ TO QUAKER LAKE, ASP 3, AND 280

that are more akin to small villages than typical park facilities. Indeed, this seems to have been the logic behind dividing the park into two sections, as the Red House and Quaker areas are the two hubs of development. The colonies of cabins often resemble neighborhoods on the fringes of each village's cluster of stores, museums, and dining and recreational venues.

Because the park is so large, bringing a bike (rentals are available) is a good idea. Miles of hiking trails allow campers to explore the mixed-hardwood forests, mountains, streams, and ponds. Two artificial lakes offer swimming at sandy beaches and boating activities. To ensure quiet, calm waters, boating is limited to nonmotorized craft or boats with only small motors. Visitors who wish to gain a deeper understanding of the park's history and natural features can join the park staff and naturalists on structured tours, walks, or similar activities. The park is open year-round—numerous winterized cabins visitors allow exploration of this wilderness by ski, snowshoe, or snowmobile.

GETTING THERE

From Interstate 86, take Exit 18, NY 280. Head south on NY 280 for 4.4 miles. Park entrance is straight ahead.

GPS COORDINATES

PARK ENTRANCE:

UTM Zone (WGS84) 17T
Easting 675981
Northing 4657022
Latitude N 42°02'44"
Longitude W 78°52'25"

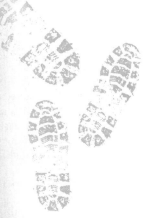

> *Sites along the middle of Loops A, B, C, and D lie very close to the lake, and the sounds of water lapping on its rocky shore are particularly pleasant here.*

THE **GREAT LAKES CONTAINS** 20 percent of the world's surface fresh water. Besides the implications of this fact, the lakes continually influence the region's environment through lake-effect rain and snow—a constant source of grumbling in central New York. Within the immediate vicinity of the Great Lakes, winds blowing off the lakes create a more favorable environment for agriculture—which explains why the southern shores of Lake Ontario contain some of New York's most productive fruit orchards. Nestled among these orchards is Lakeside Beach State Park. In fact, up until 1962, when the state established the 743-acre park, it was farmland and fruit orchards.

The campground is laid out in seven one-way loops, with the first four bordering Lake Ontario. The loops in this pet-free area (A, B, C, and D) are laid out roughly the same and share similar characteristics. The first and last couple of sites along each of these loops lie on an open lawn, which leaves campers plenty of room to spread out but not much privacy. The forested areas have a dense tree canopy as well as shrubs, saplings, and other vegetation, which enhances the woodland feel and increases privacy as well. The amply sized sites are a little closely spaced, but the understory prevents the area from feeling crowded. Sites along the middle of the loops lie very close to the lake, and the sounds of water lapping on its rocky shore are particularly pleasant here. Although many of the park's sites are similar, campers will want to take note of some differences. For example, Loop A is wooded only along its initial third (sites 4 through 13). The rest of the sites lie on an open lawn with only a few shade trees interspersed. Though these sites lack the seclusion characteristic of those in the forest, they do have the benefit of fine views of the lake. Although sites in the loop's center and closer to its end have poor views, those at the lake's edge (14 through 23) have truly expansive views of Lake Ontario. Clearly, the peripheral sites are the primary choice along this loop.

RATINGS

Beauty: ☆ ☆ ☆
Privacy: ☆ ☆ ☆
Quiet: ☆ ☆ ☆
Cleanliness: ☆ ☆ ☆
Security: ☆ ☆ ☆
Spaciousness: ☆ ☆ ☆

Along the other loops, the views of the lake, where available, are generally thinly veiled by the surrounding forest—though this is really an enhancement rather than detraction. On Loop B, views of the lake begin around site 19 and conclude around site 28—these are also some of the best sites in the whole campground. On Loop C, Lake Ontario reveals itself around site 17 and disappears around site 28. On Loop D, the lake becomes visible around site 7 because of a neighboring lawn and playing field; the views become really magnificent around site 12 but then decline at site 20, where the thick woodlands come to dominate the landscape. Sites beside the lawn are a little less private, since the forest is fairly thin—but the added views are fair compensation. Whether forested or open, sites in this part of the campground provide sounds and smells of the lake that are particularly appealing.

The next area, which includes all of the loops that allow pets (E through G), lies across the road from the park store, laundry, recreation hall, and playfield. Loop E begins and ends with seven sites (1 through 4, 39 through 41) that have views of Lake Ontario down and across the playfield. These spacious lawn sites are wide open, with no shade. Dense conifers and shrubs to the south and east enclose this section, which ends after site 22, where the loop enters the forest. Within the forest, the sites have less understory, so there is more room to spread out than in the previous forested sites bordering the lake. Also, the woodland sites have a more open-woodland feel, as beech and its telltale thickets become the dominant species. Loop E reverts to a lawn setting at site 38, but more woodland sites are available along Loop F.

All of the sites on Loop F are within forest, with the exception of 23 through 31, which are on a lawn. Glimpses of Lake Ontario are available from sites 1, 3, 5, and 6, making these scenic choices for pet owners whose choices are limited to these loops. Loop G is composed entirely of wide-open lawn sites exactly like those along Loop E, only without lake views.

Although there is no swimming beach or boat launch within the park, the lakeside setting nevertheless provides an excellent camping choice. Visitors who wish to boat on Lake Ontario can launch at Oak Orchard State Park, a short drive east along Orchard

KEY INFORMATION

ADDRESS: Route 18 Waterport, NY 14571

OPERATED BY: New York State Office of Parks, Recreation and Historic Preservation

INFORMATION: (315) 947-5205; nysparks.state.ny.us

OPEN: Late April–late October

SITES: 274 tent sites, all electric

EACH SITE HAS: Picnic table and fire ring

ASSIGNMENT: Choose from available sites or reservations

REGISTRATION: 3 p.m.–9 p.m.

FACILITIES: Picnic areas, potable water, flush toilets, park store, laundry, showers

PARKING: At site

FEE: $13/night most tent sites; add $3/night Friday, Saturday, and holidays

ELEVATION: 289 feet

RESTRICTIONS: *Pets:* Limited to Loops E, F, and G; dogs on leash with proof of currently valid rabies vaccination.
Fires: In fire rings only
Alcohol: Allowed
Vehicles: RVs and trailers allowed
Other: Quiet hours 10 p.m.–7 a.m.; 6 people maximum/ site; maximum 14-night stay
Reservations: 2-night stay required

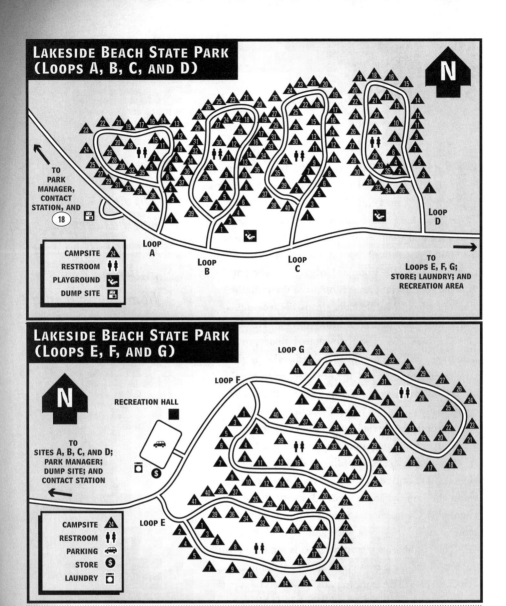

LAKESIDE BEACH STATE PARK (LOOPS A, B, C, AND D)

N

TO
PARK
MANAGER,
CONTACT
STATION, AND
(18)

CAMPSITE
RESTROOM
PLAYGROUND
DUMP SITE

LOOP
A

LOOP
B

LOOP
C

LOOP
D

TO
Loops E, F, G;
STORE; LAUNDRY; AND
RECREATION AREA

LAKESIDE BEACH STATE PARK (LOOPS E, F, AND G)

N

RECREATION HALL

TO
SITES A, B, C, AND D;
PARK MANAGER;
DUMP SITE; AND
CONTACT STATION

LOOP G

LOOP F

LOOP E

CAMPSITE
RESTROOM
PARKING
STORE
LAUNDRY

GETTING THERE

From I-90 (New York State Thruway), take Exit 48, NY 98/Batavia. Head north along NY 98 toward Albion and continue for 24 miles. Merge straight ahead onto NY 18, follow for 2.5 miles, and then turn right onto Lakeside Beach Road. The park entrance is straight ahead.

Creek. Camping registration gives you access to this boat launch. Excellent fishing is available along the creek and in Lake Ontario.

GPS COORDINATES

UTM Zone (WGS84)	17T
Easting	723963
Northing	4805245
Latitude	N 43°22'00"
Longitude	W 78°14'09"

50
LETCHWORTH
STATE PARK

THE MAJESTIC CANYON HERE has been cut by the Genesee River over millennia as it runs north from Pennsylvania to Lake Ontario. Throughout the park, dramatic views of the sheer sandstone and shale walls, some of which rise more than 600 feet, are visible from numerous scenic overlooks and along the popular Gorge Trail. The park's three large waterfalls are visible from the trail, the tallest of which, Middle Falls, drops 107 feet and is illuminated each night from May through October.

The park is very well developed, thanks to its namesake, William Pryor Letchworth, who originally purchased 190 acres and then proceeded to acquire more land and develop the area so that the public could easily enjoy this natural wonder. Extensive construction was carried out by the Civilian Conservation Corps, which expanded upon the infrastructure. A truly striking example of the work done here is the arched stone bridge that crosses the Genesee River below the Lower Falls at a very dramatic flume. The Highbanks Camping Area and swimming pools are some of the more recent and significant additions.

The Highbanks Camping Area is separated from the rest of the park by a check-in area that limits vehicle access. The camping area is served by a park store, laundry, recreation building, ball field, and playground. Every site has a minimum 20-amp hookup.

The campground is divided into several one-way loops that run parallel to each other within their respective groups. Loops 100 and 200 form one group, whereas Loops 300 through 600 and Loops 700 and 800 form their own groups. Each loop has comfort stations with showers, a recycling station, and a dumpster.

Loop 100 is the farthest from the others and consequently offers a bit more quiet and privacy. Generally, the sites are roomy, with shrubs and saplings

> *The majestic canyon here has been cut by the Genesee River over millennia as it runs from Pennsylvania to Lake Ontario.*

RATINGS

Beauty: ✿ ✿
Privacy: ✿ ✿ ✿
Quiet: ✿ ✿
Cleanliness: ✿ ✿ ✿
Security: ✿ ✿ ✿ ✿ ✿
Spaciousness: ✿ ✿ ✿

ADDRESS: 1 Letchworth
State Park
Castile, NY 14427

OPERATED BY: New York State
Office of Parks,
Recreation and His-
toric Preservation

INFORMATION: (585)-237-3303;
nysparks.state.ny.us

OPEN: Mid-May–
mid-October

SITES: 270 tent sites, 270
electric sites

EACH SITE HAS: Picnic table and
fire ring

ASSIGNMENT: Choose from
available sites or
reservations

REGISTRATION: 3 p.m.–9 p.m.

FACILITIES: Picnic areas, pavilion, potable water,
flush toilets, show-
ers, laundry, ball
field, playgrounds,
pool, museum, inn
and restaurant

PARKING: At site

FEE: $13/night most tent
sites; add $3/night
Friday, Saturday,
and holidays

ELEVATION: 919 feet

RESTRICTIONS: *Pets:* Limited to
Loops 100, 200, and
700 only; dogs on
leash with proof of
currently valid
rabies vaccination
Fires: In fire rings
only
Alcohol: Allowed
Vehicles: 1 RV or
trailer/site
Other: Quiet hours
10 p.m.–7 a.m.;
6 people maximum/
site; maximum
14-night stay
Reservations: 2-night
stay required

partially masking them from view. The exterior sites at the beginning of Loop 100 neighbor sites on Loop 200, but sites farther along Loop 100's outer edge blend into the hardwood forest. The inner sites along this loop are more spacious but have less cover, with the last few situated essentially upon an open lawn.

Loop 200 lies next to the playground, with a sparse understory offering little privacy for the initial edge sites. These grassy sites are denser, have less shade, and are openly visible to each other. The south-ern edge of this loop offers the most privacy, with ample shade from the forest canopy. The last few sites along the edge of Loop 200 abut the road, and open-ings in the understory reveal vehicle traffic as well as bike and foot traffic heading to the trailheads near the beginning of Loop 100.

Loops 300, 400, 500, and 600 are all very similar to each other: they are all roughly elongated ovals running from their entrances on their western end toward undisturbed forests to the east. The ellipses are essentially parallel, so that sites along the longer sides back up to one another. Consequently, sites at the east-ern end are the most spacious and private, and there-fore most desirable. Generally speaking, the interior sites are smaller, less shaded, and more public, as they are usually closest to the central comfort station. All of the sites would be considered in the forest and have increasing amounts of shade the farther you get from the interior of these loops.

Loop 300 borders the ball field; sites on the loop's northern edge are on an open lawn beside the field, and so are highly visible to the public. On Loop 400, sites are generally more spacious and shady and have some understory between them, which makes them a little more private than others within this group. On Loop 500, sites have fewer shrubs than on previous loops, but many are also shadier and have grassy areas. The last loop, 600, is separated from the steep banks along its southern edge by a chain-link fence. Its sites are more removed from the public areas of the campground and have only one neighboring loop, but a lack of shrubs makes them more visible to each other than on other loops.

MAP

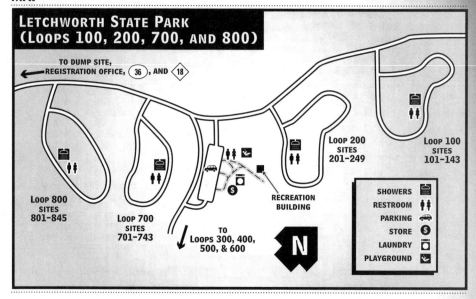

LETCHWORTH STATE PARK (LOOPS 100, 200, 700, AND 800)

TO DUMP SITE,
REGISTRATION OFFICE, 36, AND 18

LOOP 200
SITES
201–249

LOOP 100
SITES
101–143

LOOP 800
SITES
801–845

LOOP 700
SITES
701–743

TO
LOOPS 300, 400,
500, & 600

RECREATION
BUILDING

SHOWERS	
RESTROOM	
PARKING	
STORE	
LAUNDRY	
PLAYGROUND	

N

Loops 700 and 800 are closest to the campground entrance and have some of the largest sites. These loops are also composed of elongated ovals running parallel to each other, though in this case their orientation is north–south, with entrances to the north and woods to the south. Not surprisingly, the south end is the shadiest and most spacious. The long sides of Loop 700 are visible either to Loop 800 or to the road that provides access to the previous group. Multiple sites on Loop 700 are lawn sites and have 50-amp hookups, so the area is best suited to large RVs. Sites on Loop 800 are similar to those on Loop 700 in that they are deep and seem suited to RVs. However, sites along the southern edge of Loop 800 border the woods, enjoy plenty of shade, and have a lush understory.

The park's developed areas include numerous picnic grounds as well as two swimming pools, cabins, a lodge, an inn, a restaurant, concession stands, a museum, and several historic sites. Winding roads lead you through beautiful hardwood forests crisscrossed by hiking trails. Private outfitters within the park's boundaries offer daily hot-air-balloon rides along the river, horseback riding, and canoeing and rafting trips.

GETTING THERE

From I-90 (New York State Thruway), take Exit 46, I-390 South/Corning. Follow I-390 for 27.2 miles to Exit 7, NY 408/Mount Morris/Letchworth State Park. Turn left onto NY 408/Mount Morris Geneseo Road; follow 1.8 miles. Turn right on NY 36/Main Street; go north for 1.1 miles. Park entrance is on left.

GPS COORDINATES

PARK ENTRANCE:
UTM Zone (WGS84)	18T
Easting	263401
Northing	4736041
Latitude	N 42°44'25"
Longitude	W 77°53'26"

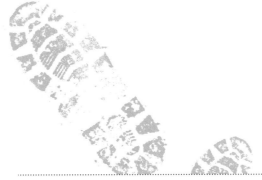

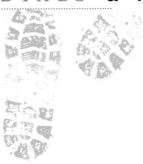

APPENDIXES & INDEX

APPENDIX A:
CAMPING-EQUIPMENT
CHECKLIST

Except for the large and bulky items on this list, we keep a plastic storage container full of the essentials for car camping, so they're ready to go when we are. We make a last-minute check of the inventory, resupply anything that's low or missing, and away we go.

COOKING UTENSILS
Bottle opener
Bottles of salt, pepper, spices, sugar, cooking oil, and maple syrup in waterproof, spillproof containers
Can opener
Cups, plastic or tin
Dish soap (biodegradable), sponge, and towel
Flatware
Food of your choice
Frying pan
Fuel for stove
Matches in waterproof container
Plates
Pocketknife
Pot with lid
Spatula
Stove
Tin foil
Wooden spoon

FIRST-AID KIT
See Introduction, pages 5–6, for a complete list.

SLEEPING GEAR
Pillow
Sleeping bag
Sleeping pad, inflatable or insulated
Tent with ground tarp and rainfly

MISCELLANEOUS
Bath soap (biodegradable), washcloth, and towel
Camp chair
Candles
Cooler
Deck of cards
Fire starter
Flashlight with fresh batteries
Foul-weather clothing
Maps (road, topographic, trails, etc.)
Paper towels
Plastic zip-top bags
Sunglasses
Toilet paper
Trowel (for burying solid waste)
Water bottle
Wool blanket

OPTIONAL
GPS
Cell phone
Barbecue grill
Binoculars
Books on bird, plant, and wildlife identification
Fishing rod and tackle
Hatchet
Lantern

APPENDIX B:
SOURCES OF INFORMATION

ADIRONDACK MOUNTAIN CLUB
814 Goggins Road
Lake George, NY 12845
(518) 668-4447
www.adk.com

ADIRONDACK REGIONAL TOURISM COUNCIL
P.O. Box 2149
Plattsburgh, NY 12901
(518) 846-8016
www.visitadirondacks.com

APPALACHIAN MOUNTAIN CLUB
5 Joy Street
Boston, MA 02108
(617) 523-0636
www.outdoors.org

APPALACHIAN TRAIL CONSERVANCY
799 Washington Street
P.O. Box 807
Harpers Ferry, WV 25425-0807
(304) 535-6331
www.appalachiantrail.org

CATSKILL MOUNTAIN CLUB
P.O. Box 558
Pine Hill, NY 12465
www.catskillmountainclub.org

FINGER LAKES TRAIL CONFERENCE
6111 Visitor Center Road
Mt. Morris, NY 14510
(585) 658-9320
www.fingerlakestrail.org

NATIONAL PARK SERVICE– FIRE ISLAND NATIONAL SEASHORE
120 Laurel Street
Patchogue, NY 11772-3596
(631) 289-4810
www.nps.gov/fiis

NEW YORK STATE DEPARTMENT OF ECONOMIC DEVELOPMENT–NEW YORK STATE TOURISM
(800) 225-5697
www.iloveny.com

NEW YORK STATE DEPARTMENT OF ENVIRONMENTAL CONSERVATION
625 Broadway
Albany, NY 12233
www.dec.state.ny.us

APPENDIX B:
SOURCES OF
INFORMATION

NEW YORK STATE OFFICE OF PARKS, RECREATION AND HISTORIC PRESERVATION
Empire State Plaza
Agency Building 1
Albany NY, 12238
(518) 474-0456
nysparks.state.ny.us

NEW YORK WINE & GRAPE FOUNDATION
800 South Main Street, Suite 200
Canandaigua, NY 14424
(585) 394-3620
www.newyorkwines.org

NORTH COUNTRY TRAIL ASSOCIATION
229 East Main Street
Lowell, MI 49331
(866) 445-3628
www.northcountrytrail.org

NORTHERN FOREST CANOE TRAIL
P.O. Box 565
Waitsfield, VT 05673
(802) 496-2285
www.northernforestcanoetrail.org

RESERVEAMERICA
(800) 456-2267
www.reserveamerica.com

SEAWAY TRAIL
P.O. Box 660
Sackets Harbor, NY 13685
(315) 646-1000
www.seawaytrail.com

SUFFOLK COUNTY DEPARTMENT OF PARKS, RECREATION AND CONSERVATION
Montauk Highway
P.O. Box 144
West Sayville, NY 11796
(631) 854-4949
www.suffolkcountyny.gov

APPENDIX C:
SUGGESTED READING
AND REFERENCE

Bailey, Bill. *New York State Parks: A Complete Outdoor Recreation Guide*. Glovebox Books of America, 1997.

Burdick, Neal S. (Series Editor). *Guide to Adirondack Trails* (Volumes 1–7). Adirondack Mountain Club, 1993–2004.

Cooper, James Fenimore. *The Leatherstocking Tales* (Volumes 1 and 2). Library of America, 1995.

Ehling, William. *50 Hikes in Central New York*. Countryman Press, 1995.

Ehling, William. *50 Hikes in Western New York*. Countryman Press, 1990.

Folwell, Elizabeth. *The Adirondack Book*. Berkshire House Publishers, 2003.

Hartman, Gary. *The Campgrounds of New York*. New Country Books, 1997.

Irving, Washington. *History, Tales, and Sketches*. Library of America, 1983.

Kick, Peter. *Catskill Mountain Guide*. Appalachian Mountain Club, 2002.

Lewis, Tom. *The Hudson: A History*. Yale University Press, 2005.

McKibbon, Bill. *Wandering Home: A Long Walk Across America's Most Hopeful Landscape, Vermont's Champlain Valley and New York's Adirondacks*. Crown Books, 2005.

McMartin, Barbara. *50 Hikes in the Adirondacks*. Countryman Press, 2003.

Ostertag, Rhonda and George. *Hiking New York*. Falcon Press Publishing Company, 1996.

Schneider, Paul. *Adirondacks: A History of America's First Wilderness*. Owl Books, 1998.

Trails Illustrated. *Adirondack Park Maps* (numbers 742–746). National Geographic.

Van Diver, Bradford B. *Roadside Geology of New York*. Mountain Press Publishing Company, 1985.

INDEX

THE BEST
IN TENT
CAMPING
NEW YORK STATE

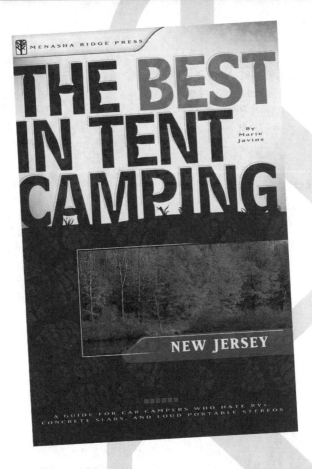

BEST IN TENT CAMPING: NEW JERSEY

by Marie Javins

ISBN 10: 0-89732-596-6
ISBN 13: 978-0-89732-596-7
$14.95; 208 pages

Camping along the Delaware River or beneath the Pine Barrens is an experience not to be missed. This book will guide you to the quietest, most beautiful, most secure campgrounds in the state.

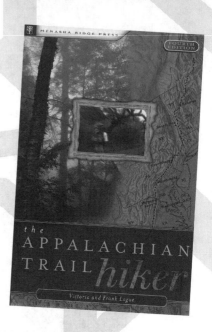
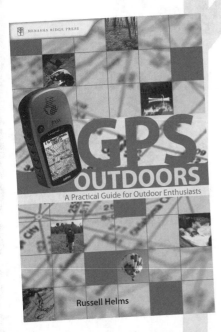

DEAR CUSTOMERS AND FRIENDS,

SUPPORTING YOUR INTEREST IN OUTDOOR ADVENTURE, travel, and an active lifestyle is central to our operations, from the authors we choose to the locations we detail to the way we design our books. Menasha Ridge Press was incorporated in 1982 by a group of veteran outdoorsmen and professional outfitters. For 25 years now, we've specialized in creating books that benefit the outdoors enthusiast.

Almost immediately, Menasha Ridge Press earned a reputation for revolutionizing outdoors- and travel-guidebook publishing. For such activities as canoeing, kayaking, hiking, backpacking, and mountain biking, we established new standards of quality that transformed the whole genre, resulting in outdoor-recreation guides of great sophistication and solid content. Menasha Ridge continues to be outdoor publishing's greatest innovator.

The folks at Menasha Ridge Press are as at home on a white-water river or mountain trail as they are editing a manuscript. The books we build for you are the best they can be, because we're responding to your needs. Plus, we use and depend on them ourselves.

We look forward to seeing you on the river or the trail. If you'd like to contact us directly, join in at www.trekalong.com or visit us at www.menasharidge.com. We thank you for your interest in our books and the natural world around us all.

SAFE TRAVELS,

Bob Sehlinger

BOB SEHLINGER
PUBLISHER

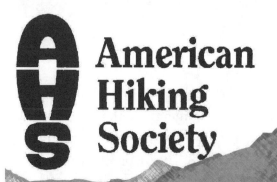
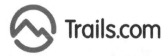
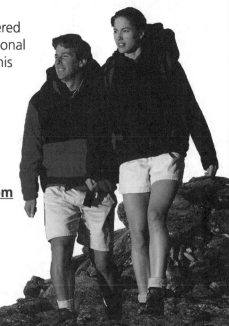